HAS HEART DISEASE
BEEN CURED ?

To Janet + Keith

[signature]

Also by Douglas Mulhall:

Our Molecular Future:
How Nanotechnology, Robotics,
Genetics, and Artificial Intelligence
Will Transform Our World

HAS HEART DISEASE BEEN CURED?

Douglas Mulhall with Katja Hansen

Foreword by
Benedict S. Maniscalco, M.D., F.A.C.C.

The Writers' Collective   Cranston, Rhode Island

Has Heart Disease Been Cured?

Douglas Mulhall with Katja Hansen

Copyright © 2003 Mulhall Hansen
Cover design by Samantha Wall
Interior design by Gene Day and Katja Hansen

ISBN, print ed.   1-932133-73-9
Printed in the United States of America
10 9 8 7 6 5 4 3 2 1

E-Mail: Order@calcify.com
Companion website: http://www.calcify.com

Library of Congress Cataloging-in-Publication Data

Mulhall, Douglas.
 Has heart disease been cured? / by Douglas Mulhall with Katja Hansen.
   p. cm.
Includes bibliographical references and index.
 ISBN 1-932133-73-9 (alk. paper)
1. Coronary heart disease—Etiology. 2. Coronary heart
disease—Treatment. 3. Coronary arteries—Infections. 4. Coronary
arteries—Calcification. I. Hansen, Katja, 1966- II. Title.
 RC685.C6M855 2003
 616.1'23—dc21   2003008085

Published by:
The Writers' Collective—Cranston, Rhode Island

For heart patients such as
the late great Douglas Adams,
who wrote *Hitchhiker's Guide to the Galaxy*,
and who died unexpectedly from a condition
that may now be detectable and preventable.

TABLE OF CONTENTS

Note on Language

Although plain language is used in this book, the topic still demands technical terms, so an easy-to-read glossary is included to explain them.

We refer often to the term *calcification*. Experts use it to describe calcium deposits in geology or medicine, but our focus is on the abnormal deposits of calcium that occur in disease. This process is known as *pathological calcification*, and for convenience we use the short form, calcification.

We also often use the term *nanobacteria*. Researchers gave this name to a special group of submicroscopic organisms. Nanobacteria are still mysterious in many ways and may not be bacteria at all. They straddle the line between life and the chemical soup in which life is created. Researchers found nanobacteria when they examined calcified deposits from the human body. They also found them in geological formations and water. Due to differing views on what they are, they have been variously referred to as "organisms," "pathogens," "bacteria-like life forms," "slime," "biofilm," and less specifically "artifacts," "vesicles," "objects," "entities," and "agents." There is still confusion over which of those descriptions is accurate. A related term, *Nanobacterium sanguineum*, (blood nanobacteria) is used by its discoverers—and in this book—to describe something that has been found in the human body. The term has been submitted for recognition to scientific journals that are regarded as the "official" repositories of species names.

This book touches on the controversy over what nanobacteria might be, but its main focus is on what they do to us and how to reverse their negative impacts.

Disclaimer

This book examines the discovery of an infectious trigger for heart disease, and a prescription drug that has been developed to reverse the impacts of a devastating illness. The text is written in plain language. It is not intended as medical guidance and should not be substituted for a physician's advice. Questions about the treatments described here should be referred to a knowledgeable practitioner. The treatments may have changed depending on when this book is being read. The authors based their work on information from patients, researchers, prescribing physicians, critics, and the drug compound developer. However, we the writers are not physicians. Many patients who have been treated for what seems to be a newly discovered trigger for heart disease are—according to their physicians—improving. On the other hand, independent studies into how quickly and consistently they improve have only just begun or are in the process of being published. Therefore these are early days. Despite this, we feel obliged to describe what is known now, and what still remains to be discovered, so that patients—especially those who have no other options—are able to ask their physicians and make their own decisions based on recommendations of their doctors. Every individual has different conditions that may or may not be addressed by such treatments. Each individual should seek qualified medical attention prior to deciding for or against every therapy.

Foreword

by Benedict S. Maniscalco, M.D., F.A.C.C.

"Miracles happen *NOT* in opposition to nature, but in opposition to what we *KNOW* of nature."

— St. Augustine

I am a reformed invasive cardiologist who used to specialize in invasive procedures for diagnosing and treating diseases of the heart and blood vessels. I founded a major heart institute in Tampa, Florida. After thirty years, when the ravages of wearing a lead apron took their toll, I decided to stop.

In all those years of doing invasive cardiology, I was clearly being a reactive physician. I was reacting to illness in patients who have late stage cardiovascular disease that is commonly known as "heart disease" or "atherosclerosis." So when I left the laboratory and shredded the lead apron, I decided to take a new look at the primary causes and potential preventions of cardiovascular disease. I got very interested in how atherosclerosis develops. In that process I learned many things more clearly than I had earlier.

The nature of atherosclerosis has eluded us for over two hundred years. We have known for at least that long that it was an inflammatory disease, but never understood why and how it begins.

I have been looking at coronary arteries for many years. Like most cardiologists, when I did an angiogram (a photograph of arteries injected with dye), if I saw no narrowing of the outline of the arteries, then I said that the coronary arteries were normal. How wrong my associates and I have been for so long!

In autopsy studies teenagers and even children ages three and four, who have died of other causes, have been shown to have the early signs of atherosclerosis in the form of fatty streaks. Moreover, a new technology called Intravascular Ultrasound (IVUS) has been used to look at the arteries of donor hearts for transplant patients. This revealed that in those hearts, which we accepted as being free of disease, there was in fact significant disease.

More importantly we've come to understand that this process is not isolated in the coronary arteries, but occurs throughout the arterial system in the body. In the natural course of the development of atherosclerosis there is a deposition of fibrous tissue, cholesterol, cellular components, chemicals and calcium in the wall of the arteries. What interests me is that the calcium is scattered throughout this collection of cellular material and is in multiple locations. Throughout the body these "deposits" occur or are in various stages of development.

I've been looking at calcium in the coronary arteries all of my professional career and never really understood how it got there. I was taught, as were most cardiologists, that calcium is part of the inflammatory response. Inflammation is the reparative response to an injury in the body's tissues. We were taught that calcium is brought to this location to repair, reinforce, and seal off the area of injury. Yet as we look at that concept, we have to ask ourselves why in the world would the body deposit calcium—the stuff that bone is made of—in its own arteries? What good would it do?

For the past generation there has been intensive investigation into the process of inflammation and the role that infectious agents might play in the inflammatory process. It is well documented in the laboratory that various viruses and bacteria can produce the inflammatory process leading to atherosclerosis. However, recent antibiotic treatments for such identified pathogens have not shown any effect on the course of the disease. In fact, there has been no statistically significant difference in the outcomes with regard to sudden death or heart attacks. Antibiotic therapy against those pathogens was ineffective.

The questions then become: What could be causing the disease that begins in childhood but does not manifest itself until the fourth, fifth, and sixth decades, and is it associated with both acute and chronic inflammation? Where did the calcium come from and why does the calcium become more and more dense?

Many of these questions are addressed in this book. Others remain unanswered. We still have a lot to learn, as the authors are correct to point out.

In introducing readers to the book, I can give this explanation as to why such a work is worthwhile to read, especially at this important juncture in medical history:

Recently my colleagues and I completed a clinical trial in which we treated patients with atherosclerosis with a new compounded prescription nanobiotic, invented and developed by Dr. Gary Mezo, to determine its impact on the pathogen *Nanobacterium sanguineum* that was discovered by Dr. Olavi Kajander and further characterized by his colleague Dr. Neva Çiftçioglu. Though our results are not yet published, the following statements can be made and will be better understood by readers once they have read this book:

✧ We can demonstrate reversal of calcium scores.

✧ Indicators of good and bad cholesterol are improving.

✧ Blood serology confirms the presence of the pathogen, while inflammation markers rise and fall as we correspondingly expose and kill it.

✧ We can demonstrate increased functional capacity in patients, along with decreased symptoms.

Whether final outcomes will change is not yet known. Like many preliminary studies, this will require another long-term study identifying all the factors that will allow us to conclude that *Nanobacterium sanguineum* is the pathogen that "triggers" the inflammatory process of atherosclerosis and pathologic calcification throughout the body. However, it is my belief that *Nanobacterium sanguineum* is the pathogen that plays this critical role in cardiovascular disease.

Finally, the new nanobiotic therapy is effective and perhaps will give us the opportunity to propose a "unifying theory of atherogenesis."

If we think that this is important today, then consider the possibilities for tomorrow. Today there is an epidemic of obesity, not just in the technologically advanced nations, but also in developing countries. This is accelerating the process of atherosclerosis, especially through the development of insulin resistance and diabetes among those who are overweight. If we don't do something about it, then tomorrow this new epidemic will do something horrendous to our record of the past twenty years in which we've reduced the number of fatal heart attacks. Instead, we will see a whole new group of patients who have aggressive and early heart disease.

The cardiovascular monster called atherosclerosis is not only ravaging our older population; it is also gathering force in the dark recesses of our children's arteries. We have much to do in just a few years to protect them. I am certain that this book will help everybody to see that there is more than just hope for a solution.

It is fortunate that the discoverers of *Nanobacterium sanguineum* chose to look at "what we know of nature" in a different way.

Benedict S. Maniscalco

Introduction

I t is time to get rid of heart disease.

This enemy has stalked us for millennia, as shown by its presence in ancient mummies. Yet it erupted as a relentless scourge only in the last century. Its tentacles now reach everywhere, afflicting at least half a billion of us on this Earth. The costs of battling its effects are gutting the budgets of families, companies, and governments. It is typically fatal, regardless of how well or early we treat it.

Happily though, if the discoveries that are described in this book hold true, then we may finally prevail.

Until now, many theories have been offered for how to cure "hardening of the arteries,"[1] but no one has given proof in an independently verified clinical trial. The quest has been haunted by a triple curse. Firstly, no published methods have reversed the fatal combination of inflammation, clotting, and buildup in blood vessels. Some drugs and diets may slow them, but none sustainably reverses them. Next, no one has shown why calcium ends up in the wrong places, causing arteries to stiffen and organs to malfunction. Finally, signs of infection keep popping up repeatedly, but no contagious "smoking gun" has been found. Possible culprits, yes. Convicted criminals, no.

This helps to explain why *half of fatal heart attacks occur with no apparent prior symptoms.*[2] The other half are treated but not fixed. Doctors and drug companies continue to care for the symptoms instead of the cause of the most prevalent terminal disease in existence.[3]

Due to this frustrating history, every new book that discusses a potential cure is bound to be met with great hope by many, and equal skepticism by researchers.

With that in mind, we knew that we'd have to be clear about who might benefit from this book, and why.

What is "evidence"?

According to the cardiologists and patients interviewed by us, thousands of heart disease victims are showing clinical signs of improvement when treated with a novel prescription drug compound aimed at a newly discovered infectious trigger for atherosclerosis. Not every patient is improving. Yet many are.

In this case, "clinical signs" means measurable evidence based on direct observation of a patient by a qualified physician. Clinical evidence is different from hearsay or "anecdotal" evidence such as "I feel better." Clinical evidence includes quantifiable measurements such as blood and other factors. These indicators are central to this book, and are explained further in the glossary at the back, under the term "clinical evidence."

In examining such preliminary reports, we as authors faced a classic dilemma: Should we write about tests and a treatment whose effectiveness has been observed, yet is still to be confirmed in exhaustive clinical studies? Or should we keep quiet until the situation is more certain?

Beneath this lies a persistent controversy over the right of very ill patients to know what new options might be open to them when apparently none are left.

With this in mind, some stark realities compelled us to go ahead.

"Too far gone?"

Millions of seriously ill heart patients have exhausted other treatments. They have already used the available surgical, drug, and "alternative" options. They are considered too far gone by most physicians to be saved from a slow decline to the grave. Describing new possibilities for this group was one of our main motivations. On one hand, we did not want to offer false hope. On the other, experience with a new approach might help such patients. That experience is not ours, but instead comes from observations by physicians who have treated patients.

The calcium mystery

We also realized that a far wider group of readers might benefit, but to show who they are we had to explore something known as "pathological calcification."

Many of us think of calcium as a good thing that is found in bones, teeth, or vitamin supplements. Yet there is a dark side to the calcium story. Most everyone over the age of fifty suffers from, or knows somebody who suffers from pathological calcification. Most patients haven't heard about it because doctors haven't known the cause. The topic is usually reserved for medical journals instead of the popular media.

Because calcification is one of the great unexplained epidemics, we saw that it was time for someone to spell out—in plain terms—*how we calcify and why it matters.*

Here we focus on calcification in heart disease because much of the early clinical evidence comes from heart patients and their physicians. Yet as we'll see, research has also been done on calcification in the kidneys, brain, tendons, prostate, and other areas of the body.

Why focus on one treatment?

Drugs known as nanobiotics are not the only chemicals that can get at calcification or its underlying trigger, but so far there is only one compound that seems to work *effectively*, without serious side effects in most patients.

Other chemicals are too toxic, or not purpose-built to get at the trigger. Nor have methods such as diet or stress therapy shown evidence of reversing the pathogen's course, although someday perhaps they may. Therefore, we refer to such methods but do not focus on them.

The nanobiotic compound described here is not just one drug, but is instead a new combination of well known drugs. While it comprises just one daily regimen, it uses many tactics to fight a stealthy enemy. As such, there is more than one story to the evolution of this strategy.

We also highlight the nanobiotic approach due to an ages-old regulatory quirk that sets medical research apart from medical practice. This allowed one innovator to bring a treatment quickly to very ill patients. Otherwise it would still be stuck in the lab.

His team is leading the way for other reasons. Due to the pathogen's peculiar characteristics, many other researchers don't know yet how to isolate it, so they aren't yet able to aim a therapy at it. Therefore, one group that learned this first has moved ahead of the others. This struggle by scientists to find and eradicate such a culprit is one of the more remarkable detective stories in medical history, so we spend the early part of the book describing it. As other companies and researchers discover this pathway, there is no doubt that other competitive treatments will arise, and when they do, we will cover them in upcoming editions of this book.

The story is just beginning

History shows us that many drugs used today took years to emerge from obscurity. For example, antibiotics took decades to discover, were ignored when first announced, then required years of research to be produced in bulk.[4]

The situation may be similar with nanobiotics. They are based on years of discovery, and until now were unnoticed except by physicians or researchers who work with them.

Yet one difference between the first antibiotics and the first nanobiotics is that antibiotics were newly isolated chemicals aimed at a well known group of bacteria, whereas nanobiotics are well known chemicals aimed at a newly isolated pathogen in a novel way.[5] Another difference is that patients are much more educated about their medical choices now than when antibiotics were discovered.

Will such differences shorten the timeframe between discovery and widespread adoption? Hopefully so, if the treatment fulfills its early promise. But we'll see from other examples that this is not guaranteed.

We agree with researchers who developed tests and a treatment for this "trigger," and with the critics who are skeptical of it, that more study is required. In fact, more is underway. The discussion is just beginning.

We are telling the story right now so that patients, physicians, and researchers might be inspired to investigate further. This is especially true for patients who have exhausted their other treatment options.

As research proceeds, we will post updates at www.calcify.com.

PART I

WHAT GROWS
IN SO MANY OF US

CHAPTER ONE

When To Say
"I'm Cured"

Most of us are used to hearing that the successful struggle against infectious diseases has improved our lives. Yet, after a century and a half of winning more battles than we lose, the question is: Where are we in that war; near the end, the middle, or still at the beginning? Have we exhausted the list of great discoveries that enhance our longevity and provide other mass benefits, or are we about to cross another threshold?

Just a handful of remarkable innovations has been responsible for much of our good fortune. One was the discovery of a link between bacteria and infection.[1] This led to what is still one of the best disease prevention methods: Washing our hands.[2] Another was the vaccine, which controlled or eradicated infections such as smallpox, diphtheria, and tuberculosis that made humanity miserable for millennia.

Throughout the centuries[3] medical experts have theorized that heart disease[4] is also an infection, but despite this history the idea did not take hold in western medical thinking until just a few years ago. Why? Because no one had found a "smoking gun."

Today many researchers are hunting for infection in heart disease and generating hundreds of medical articles about it. Therefore it's easy to see how the discoveries described here did not spring from a miraculous or mysterious source. Instead, they came from investigations by experts into well-known fields. Just as penicillin was credited to the work of a few but depended on much work by others, so the quest for an infectious trigger in heart disease fits that pattern.

Nor is it surprising that scientists would find a heart disease trigger when we consider that billions of dollars have been devoted to researching it. However, the remarkable story is how a few innovators found a path overlooked by other researchers throughout the decades. Here we describe that path, instead of just starting with the treatment, to show why such a therapy is not an unexplained miracle. Instead, it came from a lot of work and a bit of luck. Vast areas were investigated. We'll explore how they came together in an impressive sequence of tests and treatments.

What does being "cured" mean?

In plain terms, being "cured" of an illness means getting rid of it so that it doesn't come back, then being restored to good health. This may seem obvious, but actually there are many medical definitions of a cure. These range from finding no detectable trace of an infection over a few weeks, to being free of something such as cancer over many years.[5]

We can be cured of an illness but still be stuck with the effects. This is the case with leprosy, for example, in which patients may be cured but still suffer internal or external scars. Such lingering damage must also be considered with a "cure" for heart disease.

To get rid of atherosclerosis, which is the type of heart disease that we focus on here, we first have to fix what comes with it. The earliest indicator is swelling (also known as inflammation) that narrows circulatory vessels. The next is soft and hard plaque: a gooey substance comprised of fats, fiber, and calcified deposits that many of us know as hardening of the arteries. Finally there is clotting; a normally healthy process that seems to go haywire in blocked arteries. These malfunctions are not separate, but are mixed together in a lethal combination.

Nor does a cause or cure for heart disease necessarily start with the heart. First, the tiny capillaries that make up most of our circulatory system start to plug. By the time we see a problem in the heart, those tiny veins and arteries have been sick for a while. To conquer the illness, we have to confront it at the invisible starting gate. This is why stopping it in our twenties and thirties is so vital, because the trouble starts then.

A questionable basis for treatment

The idea that most forms of cancer, heart disease, kidney stones, cataracts, and arthritis are *not* infection-related has underpinned western treatments since the mid-20th century. Most physicians, clinics, emergency rooms, hospitals, pharmacies, drug companies, and insurance plans allocate resources on the basis that these illnesses are *not* caused by infection. A good chunk of the globalized economy—in the form of a multi-trillion dollar medical industry—is based on this concept.

Because we haven't cured many of these diseases, we spend most of our resources on controlling their worst symptoms. We train medical teams to control the pain and crippling effects. Surgeons cut out or physically fix the most dangerous carnage. Pharmacists, researchers, and psychologists help us to cope with the fallout. We spend great sums on research, much of it aimed at reducing impacts. A gigantic drug and diet infrastructure is built around this. Anti-cholesterol drugs saturate our bloodstreams and permeate the advertising that surrounds us. Blood thinners, anti-stroke medicine, high blood pressure medicine, and fat-free diets are used to alleviate symptoms. Ultimately, it's an expensive, hard-fought, but losing battle. Most of us only delay the inevitable.

The depth of desperation over this was symbolized by the attention lavished worldwide on an announcement in 2003 of a "polypill" that promised to have many symptom-reducing drugs crammed into one daily pill.[6] Despite the pill not existing, not being tried, manufactured, approved, or applied to the proposed target population, the researchers claimed it would cut heart attacks by about 80 percent. While medical associations and cardiologists pointed out "massive caveats" to the untried concept of saturating the whole human population over 55 years of age with such a combination, the idea still garnered intense publicity as a potential solution; a virtually done deal.[7]

The idea is laudable for its preventative strategy, but by attacking symptoms instead of the cause it still forms part of a vast band-aid approach to a vast problem.

Treating symptoms undoubtedly helps to keep us going, but the U.S. Surgeon General says that the supporting framework—which outstrips the American military in size—is also a financial albatross around the necks of patients, businesses, and governments:

> Heart disease not only attacks our hearts; it places a burden on our healthcare system. It accounts for 29 percent of all hospitalizations, more than a third of all nursing home care, and 23 percent of hospice care. It also affects our chances of longevity. If we could eliminate heart disease, the life expectancy of the average American would increase by five years![8]

Slowing it doesn't cure it

Perhaps due to this massive investment in treating symptoms, the claim of a cure for something as basic as heart disease is often met with the same skepticism by doctors as a claim that snake oil cures gout.

In "complementary" and "alternative" medicine there are many claims about reversing heart disease. Some are based on diets, others on vitamins, and still others rely on chemically removing toxins from the blood. There is evidence that a few of these may delay or reduce the symptoms of heart disease. Yet there is no broadly accepted clinical proof to show that the blood vessel narrowing found in most heart conditions is sustainably reversed. The term "reversed" is often used in reference to heart disease diets and treatments, but close analysis reveals that this is a misstatement. Partial reversal might occur with the symptoms, but not with the cause, and usually not with the ultimate results.

It is important to distinguish between *reversing* hardening of the arteries and *slowing the rate of progression*. Drugs, diets, and surgery may retard the pace or blunt inflammation. Surgeons cut out obstructions, but these often recur. Some drug companies have specially treated tubes known as stents to prevent re-blockage of artery repairs, but these are only partially effective.[9] Whether or not they work in the long run is unknown. Drugs known as statins[10] have shown success at combating blockage, but these seem to slow rather than reverse the process.

Many physicians tell their patients that losing weight, exercising, and eating the right foods lessens the potential for heart attacks. Exactly what are the "right" foods remains open to vigorous debate.

Among the more prominent and sometimes controversial methods reported to prevent or fix heart disease are: Dr. Atkins' New Diet Revolution, The South Beach Diet,[11] Dr. Dean Ornish's Program for Reversing Heart Disease,[12] intravenous chelation therapy,[13] and the Linus Pauling unified theory of heart disease.[14] Stress management, meditation, and herbal remedies are also said to work, and are often recommended in concert with each other.

Each has its own validity. Many users swear by results. Some such therapies are also in opposition to each other.

Yet so far, no diet, drug, or therapy has succeeded in reversing everything in heart disease, including inflammation, soft and hard plaques, and fatal clotting.

The infectious culprits?

A mixed bag of viruses, bacteria, and other life-like substances occupy the deposits in our arteries at one time or another. The swollen walls of blood vessels seem to turn into garbage dumps where many pathogens thrive. Bugs such as those that cause pneumonia have been fingered as culprits.[15] Other studies have found that patients who are infected with the *Herpes simplex* virus, that causes cold sores, face a greater likelihood of heart attacks.[16] The many other suspects in heart disease are shown in Figure 1, along with brief summaries of the ailments that they are associated with.[17]

More than a few physicians believe that such infections are the primary cause. For example, some books already identify viruses and bacteria as causing coronary heart disease.[18] The trouble is evidence from clinical trial studies does not identify them to be triggers. As pointed out by Dr. Benedict Maniscalco in the Foreword to this book—and as we'll see later—no clinical trial has shown that getting rid of them *reverses* the disease.

Many pathogenic suspects have been found repeatedly at the medical crime scene and taken into custody.

Bacteroides oralis	Bacteria in gum disease
Borrelia burgdorferi	Bacterial cause of Lyme disease
Chlamydia pneumoniae	Bacteria associated with pneumonia
Coxsackievirus	Virus associated with inflammation of the heart
Cytomegalovirus	Virus that can harm individuals who have low resistance
Epstein-Barr virus	Virus associated with infectious mononucleosis and cancer
Eubacterium alactolyticum	Bacteria in gum disease
Helicobacter pylori	Bacteria associated with gastric ulcer
Hepatitis A virus	Virus associated with liver infection
Herpes Type-2 virus	Virus associated with primary genital infection and encephalitis
Mycoplasma fermentans and Mycoplasma oralis	Agent associated with gum disease
Mycoplasma genitalium	Agent associated with urogenital infection
Mycoplasma pneumoniae	Agent associated with pneumonia
Peptostreptococcus anaerobius	Bacteria in gum disease
Porphyromonas gingivalis	Bacteria in gum disease
Streptococcus sanguis and Streptococcus oralis	Bacteria in gum disease
Treponema pallidum	Bacterial cause of syphilis
Trypanozoma cruzi	Cause of Chagas disease

Figure 1: Some pathogens suspected in heart disease

Some had charges against them dismissed for lack of evidence, despite their suspicious behavior. As a group, they have yet to be tried or convicted for gang violence to the heart. They are still under surveillance.

Lessons from the stomach

Clinical trial results for treatments of these bacterial and viral infections have been disappointing,[19] but the American Heart Association notes nonetheless that researchers seem to be onto something.

> No one knows for sure what causes the low-grade inflammation that seems to put otherwise healthy people at risk. However, the new findings are consistent with the hypothesis that an infection—possibly one caused by a bacteria or a virus—might contribute to or even cause atherosclerosis....Thus, it may be that antimicrobial or antiviral therapies will someday join other therapies used to prevent heart attacks.[20]

Furthermore, the association says that a disturbing precedent should make us pay more attention:

> This idea clearly needs to be tested in clinical trials. However, the notion that chronic infection can lead to unsuspected disease isn't foreign to most doctors. For example, bacterial infection with *Helicobacter pylori* is now known to be the major cause of stomach ulcers.[21]

When someone gets an ulcer, their physician often prescribes a drug to control bacteria in their stomach that are causing the problem. The bacterium, *Helicobacter pylori,* grows in us for years without causing much trouble, but then as we age it eats away at the walls of our digestive tract. If it is left for too long, then one day we start bleeding internally from an ulcer.

For many years the solution to this was for surgeons to cut the nerve that goes from the brain to the abdomen and slice open the small intestine to get at the ulcer. It was major surgery with a painful, slow recovery.

Then in 1982 two Australian researchers, Barry Marshall and Robin Warren, discovered that *Helicobacter pylori*, a spiral-shaped bacterium, was usually present in the stomach when an ulcer occurred. This bacterium and the ulcers that it triggers are now commonly treated with antibiotics. Expensive and risky surgery is virtually never used anymore.[22]

Here is the astonishing part: Despite compelling scientific evidence and clear signs of success, *it took from the early 1980s when the treatment was developed, until the mid 1990s for the approach to gain widespread acceptance.* In that interval, according to the U.S. Center for Disease Control, vast numbers of patients were prescribed ineffective drugs or underwent painful and unnecessary surgery.

This sad history is well known to physicians and government authorities, but the question is, what has been learned? By ignoring infectious signs in heart disease, might we be committing a similar mistake?

Check your teeth

Gum disease is also mentioned frequently in Figure 1. The links between oral and cardiac health are the subject of intense scrutiny by dentists and cardiologists. Studies have drawn a close correlation between patients who've had periodontal disease and those who suffer from heart disease.[23] Some dentists have started to pay more attention to the general health of patients rather than just teeth, while some cardiologists are looking at patients' teeth instead of just the heart.

Once again, the connection wasn't just suddenly discovered. It emerged over the years as physicians and dentists began to observe that heart patients also had a history of gum disease. However, the connection has only recently started to be solidified.

Are they the cause, or just opportunistic?

Although many bacteria and viruses have been found in heart disease, it is still not clear as to *when* they take hold in the decades-long process, and whether one of them is a primary trigger or an ongoing cause. For example, some studies show no correlation between infection with such pathogens and the onset of heart disease.[24] This relatively new observation suggests that instead of being at the root of heart disease, many infections take hold at a later stage.

Other studies suggest that as time goes on, the more stress that occurs in the body from multiple infections, the worse heart disease gets.[25] This is referred to as "total pathogen load." Once the body is weakened by such infections, it is open to diseases that may gain a hold after earlier invasions have occurred. Therefore, while they may not be the triggers, infections that gang up on our heart to kill us still warrant serious attention. We don't just write off such bugs because they aren't shown to be there from the start. For example, some evaluations show that heart patients have a lower short-term recurrence of problems when treated with antibiotics.[26] This supports the idea that if we fight off infection, we might be able to fight heart disease.

Yet there is a problem. Doctors haven't *cured* heart disease just by using antibiotics. They only temporarily alleviate a few symptoms. Why don't antibiotics that normally kill these organisms reverse heart disease? Are such infections secondary to an underlying problem? Did the attackers sneak in when the body's defenses were already weakened? Or were they there from the beginning?

Another paradox is that most such pathogens grow and replicate at a fast rate that can be monitored, so how could they drive a slow process such as atherosclerosis?

Is it the same as with ulcers, where a bacterium triggers ulceration over time? Might we be continually re-infected, so that the process degrades our resistance?

Somehow, it seems that a mysterious underlying infection is causing blood vessel irritation that comes and goes throughout our lives as the body's defenses, or administered drugs, struggle in vain to kill it.

Genetics and environment

Heredity and environment also determine whether we can fight off such infections. Some of us may have natural immunity. Also, many environments are more "heart disease friendly" than others.

These factors are especially important because many persons who live a healthy lifestyle still get heart disease and die from it. Predisposition at a young age is the subject of intense genetic research. Scientists believe that they have found genes that make us more—or less—susceptible.[27] Yet such susceptibility may not be the cause. It is only a sign that some of us are programmed to be more open, or react more or less severely to that cause.

The genetic approach is not to be underestimated. Now that the human genome has been largely decoded, we can hope for remarkable discoveries about our susceptibility to many diseases.

Yet the environments where we live and work also contribute to sparking or suppressing illness. Many studies show that some diseases are concentrated in geographic clusters throughout the world. Kidney stones, some cancers, and other ailments are found in such clusters, but it is not always understood why.

Therefore, to fully exploit the benefits of environmentally and genetically related therapies, we still have to know the triggers for these illnesses.

Finding the spark

We've seen here that heart disease doesn't show up in a singular way, but rather involves thousands of chemical and biological interactions that make a cure hard to find.

That is why scientists who are investigating one special infection say that it may not be the only "cause." Instead, it is a "trigger" that activates other processes, then continues to re-activate them throughout our lives.

The greatness of the discovery may be that they have found what kick-starts, then accelerates disease in those susceptible to the trigger.

With this in mind, let's look at an insidious process known as "calcification."

CHAPTER TWO

Guess What?
You're On The Calcification List

If calcification were classified as a disease, then it would be the most widespread illness on Earth. That may seem like a bold statement, but as we'll see, there is much evidence to back it up.

Most patients have never heard of the term "calcification" because it hasn't been explained to them. It's not surprising. Most doctors don't understand why it is present or what triggers it, so they don't pay much attention to it.

The variety of terms used to describe calcification is bewildering. When those terms are assembled into one list, it is easy to see why this menace managed to stay out of the limelight. Like a charlatan, it goes by many names that mask its true role in causing trouble (see Fig. 2).

Calcification-related conditions shown in Figures 3 and 4 share at least one trait: They are "pathological." That is, they harm the human body.

Pathological calcification is not the healthy process that builds bones and teeth, but instead it is found in disease.[1]

Calcification By Many Other Names

Apatite deposits (nothing to do with "appetite")

Brain sand (calcium deposits in the brain)

Calcified deposits

Calcinogenic (causing calcification)

Calcium buildup

Calcium deposition

Calcium phosphate (chemical symbol $CaPO_4$)

Calcium salts

Calculus (stone in the kidneys, gall bladder, etc.)

Cysts (many but not all cysts are calcified)

Dystrophic calcification (hardening that results from disease occurring at the site of calcification)

Extraskeletal calcification (calcification that takes place outside bones and teeth)

Hard plaque (found in gums and arteries)

"Hardening" of various bodily systems

Metastatic calcification (results from disease occurring far from the site of calcification)

Microcalcification (often found in breast cancer)

Mineralization (also applied to other types of mineral deposits)

Ossification (deposits of bone-like material in soft tissue)

Plaque (soft and hard deposits in blood vessels)

Spurs (as in bone spurs)

Stones (such as kidney, gum, and gall stones)

Figure 2: The many faces of calcification. *These terms are used to describe calcification in disease. Each word depicts the same process; that is, formation of harmful calcium phosphate deposits in the body.*

Leading us to the heart...and into space

Such calcium deposits are found in the arteries of our heart—sometimes leading to heart attacks—and in our neck vessels—sometimes leading to stroke. They are in the cataracts that blind millions. They accumulate in the kidneys and gall bladder to form painful stones and in the gums to cause inflammation. They interfere with the brain, nerves, and glands. They are in the cells of Alzheimer's patients. They surround bone joints that are crippled by arthritis and spurs. They are well-known symptoms of breast cancer and liver cysts. They are in the cells that are afflicted by skin diseases. They invade the prostate and ovaries.

At the fringe of exploration the process afflicts astronauts who've been in space. The National Aeronautics and Space Administration (NASA) sees it as an ongoing astronaut health problem and a potential barrier to getting human beings to other planets. When astronauts go into space and after they come back home, they often are at risk of developing kidney stones, calcified coronary arteries, and arthritis "flare-ups." If astronauts are incapacitated by stones that block their urinary tracts, then space trips might have to be aborted.[2]

What happens to those astronauts is an acceleration of what happens to many of us here on Earth: Calcium deposits show up in the wrong parts of the body.

Most of us are somewhere on the calcification list. The chances are good that, if you're over forty years of age and have suffered acute aches or pains repeatedly in your muscles or joints, then you've got calcification. If you're not that old, or don't have those symptoms, then probably your friends or relatives have them.

If you're lucky enough not to be directly affected, then a good part of your income tax, sales tax, and health insurance premiums still goes to a medical system that is struggling to keep up with the havoc wreaked by diseases that are on the list.

The Calcification List

Alzheimer's (deterioration of brain function)

Arteriosclerosis and atherosclerosis (see Heart disease below)

Arthritis (osteo and rheumatoid)[3]

Autism (childhood brain disorder)

Bone spurs

Brain sand and brain cysts

Breast cancer

Bursitis (inflammation of the joints)

Calcinosis cutis (calcium deposits in the skin)

Cataracts

Deafness from middle ear ossification

Diabetes (type 2 in adults)

Eczema (skin rash often from allergic reaction)

Gall stones

Glaucoma (eye disease that degrades vision)

Heart disease, notably arteriosclerosis and atherosclerosis[4]

Heterotopic ossification (bone formation in soft tissue)

Hypoparathyroidism (low production of some hormones)

Kidney stones, cysts, Polycystic Kidney Disease (PKD)

Liver cysts

Macular degeneration (degradation of a part of the eyes)

Meniere's Disease (vertigo from inner ear malfunction)

Multiple Sclerosis (degradation of the nervous system)

Parathyroid disease (affects hormones that balance calcium)

Prostatitis (inflammation of the prostate gland)

Psoriasis (inflammation of the skin)

Salivary gland stones

Scleroderma (hardening of the skin)

Tendinitis (inflammation of tendons)

Figure 3: The calcification list. *These diseases usually contain calcification. See also Figure 4 showing where calcium associated with some of these illnesses is deposited in the human body.*

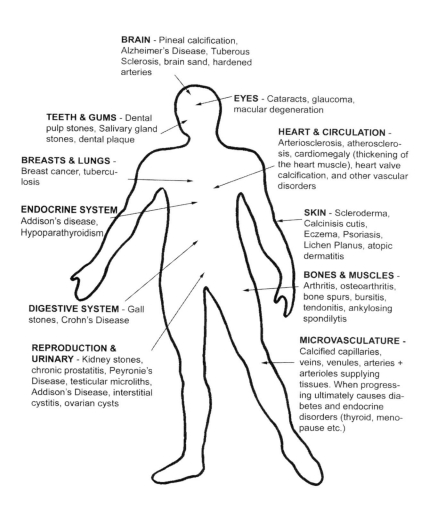

Figure 4: Some areas of calcification in the human body

To understand how important it is to find a solution, check the impressive list of diseases that contain calcium deposits where they are not supposed to be (see Fig. 3 and 4).

How to "see" the problem?

Until now the failure to solve calcification has been understandable because doctors were only able to accurately measure changes in calcified deposits in the last few years. Fast scanning methods to photograph the body in a fraction of a heartbeat are relatively new. Terms such as *CT Scan*, *EBCT*, and *Ultra Fast Scan* (see Glossary for definitions) describe progressive steps in that quest to see calcium deposits without cutting open the body.

Despite such advances, experts *still* can't see much of the accompanying inflammation in arteries without physically invading the body in a risky procedure. We'll discuss this problem further in the next chapter.

The Nasty Details

Calcification attacks us in our youth, then degrades us as we age. This insidious monster makes us miserable, then kills us. Here are explanations of some conditions that are related to calcification. Taken together, they affect most of us in one way or another. If some terms are unfamiliar, please refer to the Glossary in the back of this book.

Heart and circulation

If heart disease treatment were classified as an industry, then it would rank among the top financial sectors of the world economy. Aneurysms, arteriosclerosis, atherosclerosis, acute coronary syndrome, angina, cardiomegaly (thickening of the heart muscle), heart valve calcification, heart attack, high blood pressure (hypertension), many circulatory problems and arrhythmia, stroke, and other vascular disorders each contain calcification. Such diseases became more prevalent after World War II and have been blamed on lifestyles of the post-war era.[5] Treatments range from exercise and dietary changes to heart surgery and drug therapy. There are angioplasties—where a blocked artery is inflated for temporary relief—along with arterial stents where a metal tube is put in the artery to keep it open. In bypass surgery, veins are taken from another part of the body and put around the heart to restore blood flow. Such therapies are so prevalent now that they constitute the lifeblood of many hospitals and the drug industry.

Diabetes. This disrupts the way the body works, resulting in thirst and increased urination. Diabetes is associated with obesity and atherosclerosis in adults, but it is showing up at an alarming rate among children.[6] In diabetic patients calcification is a strong predictor of death from heart failure.[7]

Calciphylaxis. This is an extremely fast and fatal form of calcification (death occurs in one month) that may occur in patients with severe kidney diseases and with a disease of the parathyroid gland; hypoparathyroidism.[8]

Teeth and gums

More and more the condition of the mouth is seen as mirroring the condition of the body. This isn't surprising when we consider that most of what goes into us must pass through the mouth. As explained earlier, there seems to be a link between calcified deposits in the mouth and those found in arteries leading to the heart.

Salivary gland stones. These calcified stones are painful when they block glands that produce saliva.[9]

Dental calcification. It seems strange to say that calcium deposits are found around teeth, because most of us know that teeth are made of calcium. Yet this more harmful type of "pathological" calcification occurs around teeth, for example, in the form of "calculus" that occurs near and beneath the gum line.[10] Equally serious are chronic inflammation and other types of calcification that develop in the gums and jaw, leading to tooth loss. New analysis shows that the type of inflammation and clotting in tiny blood vessels around decayed teeth is remarkably similar to the clotting, or thrombosis, that happens in heart attacks and strokes.[11] Thus, there seems to be a link between calcification, inflammation, and clotting here.

Brain

Stroke. This is actually "vascular" (circulatory) disease, but its main impact is on the brain. Hardening of the arteries throughout the body leads to clots that cut off the blood supply. This leads to catastrophic loss of memory, motor function, and reasoning power. It can cause death.

Cranial calcification. Some disorders cause calcium to be deposited in the brain.[12]

Alzheimer's Disease. Among the prevalent diseases, this one is most feared by elderly persons, due to the loss of familiar personal traits and recognition abilities that accompany it. As the population lives longer, Alzheimer's afflicts a growing percentage of persons. And it doesn't start only in old age.[13] Short-circuiting of the brain plaques and neuron synapses causes memory loss and confusion, then progresses to violent outbursts and inability to function. Excesses of calcium have been found in the brain synapses of Alzheimer's patients. Because it is well known that too much calcium can lead to cell death, it is theorized that this overload kills brain cells.[14]

Tuberous Sclerosis. At the other end of the age scale is a disorder affecting newborns, which is caused by damage to genes that regulate cell growth. Its tumors affect the brain, skin, and kidneys. It is often associated with autism.[15] Not to be confused with tuberculosis (TB).

Breasts and lungs

Breast cancer. The National Cancer Institute estimates that one in eight American women will develop breast cancer in their lifetimes.[16] It is a leading cause of death among females. Men can develop the same breast cancers that occur in women, although the percentage of men who develop them is much lower. The cause of this cancer is unknown. A prime characteristic is calcified fibrous nodules.[17] Some treatments such as surgery, chemotherapy, and radiation are able to send breast cancer into remission.

Tuberculosis. TB is a bacterial infection of the lungs, which still occurs in many developing nations. Calcified nodules are commonly found in tuberculosis patients.[18]

Bones and muscles

Arthritis. This affects nearly 43 million Americans making it one of the most prevalent diseases in the United States.[19] Arthritis is a general term applied to more than a hundred different types of joint problems, most of which are characterized by inflammation and painful movement, along with abnormal calcification in and around the joints.[20] There are many therapies, but no cure.

Bone spurs. Also known as osteophytes, these are enlargements in the bony structure in the neck, back, and weight-bearing or overused areas. Ligaments calcify, causing pressure on the spine and pain during movement.[21] Injections and surgical removal are the current therapies.

Bursitis and Tendonitis. Pain and stiffening of the joints, characterized by inflammation and calcification of the bursa and tendons.[22]

Osteoporosis. This loss of bone mass affects many aging women. There seems to be a link between such loss and calcification of the arteries, where calcium may go out of bones and into the arteries, but this research is still at an early stage.[23] Treatments include drugs and vitamin supplements, although these do not cure the condition.

Ears and Balance

Meniere's Disease, Vertigo. The inner ear regulates balance with fluid. Sometimes tiny stones in the ear seem to undergo a chemical change from calcium carbonate to calcium phosphate, then roll around in the fluid, throwing us off balance.[24] The cause and cure are still unknown.

Eyes

Glaucoma, cataracts, and macular degeneration together are responsible for most age-related vision loss and blindness in persons over the age of fifty. Each is characterized by calcified buildups throughout the eye.

Glaucoma. This causes the loss of a nerve fiber layer in the eye, leading to blindness. Millions of victims are afflicted. Calcification is usually seen at the site of the problem.[25]

Cataracts. These are characterized by early presence of small, calcified particles and fibrous tissue that obscure vision in the lens of the eye.[26] It can usually be treated by surgically removing the lens, but sometimes it is inoperable.

Macular Degeneration. Affects the central part of the retina or "focus point" of the eye, causing decreased clarity and loss of central vision. There is no known prevention or cure, although treatments are available for early sufferers. Many seniors are affected.[27] Calcified nodules are often seen in the membranes of the macula.[28]

Digestive system

Crohn's Disease. This inflammation in the intestinal tract can trigger secondary calcification-related complications including arthritis, kidney stones, and gall stones.[29]

Gall stones. These stones often have a core made up of calcium carbonate or calcium phosphate mineral, therefore they are undoubtedly a main indicator of calcification.[30] Patients with gall stones can end up with liver disease due to obstruction of bile flow by stones.[31]

Glands

Addison's Disease. This affects hormone production. Calcification of the adrenal glands is a cause.[32]

Hypoparathyroidism. This hormone deficiency causes abnormal use of calcium and phosphorus by the body. It is often characterized by kidney stones, cataracts in the eyes, and calcification in the brain.[33]

Reproductive and urinary systems

Chronic Prostatitis. This painful inflammation of the prostate gland is often accompanied by calcification.[34]

Interstitial Cystitis. Chronic pain and spasm of the bladder that is usually associated with calcification and inflammation of the bladder wall.

Kidney stones. Stone formations in the kidneys. These often consist of a core of calcium carbonate or phosphate mineral.[35] They are dealt with in more depth in Chapter 5 (See subheading: "It started with the kidneys"). There are many treatments including drugs, surgery, and diet, but no cure. The occurrence rate is on the rise.

Ovarian cysts. These painful calcified cysts in the ovaries may result in a decreased ability to conceive children.

Peyronie's Disease. Calcification that sometimes forms in the penis, causing it to be crooked and painful when erect, disrupting sex life.[36] Surgical removal of calcium usually results in a shortening of the penis.

Testicular microliths. These are small, calcified stones in the testicles, also associated with cancer.[37]

Skin

Scleroderma. This inflammation and calcification of the skin causes thickening, hardening, and tightening of skin, blood vessels, and internal organs. It can last a long time and cause or be accompanied by heart, joint, and other problems. It often shows on radiographs as calcification of soft tissue. The cause is unknown although it is associated with the overproduction of a fibrous protein in the body.[38] There is no known cure.

Areas of low blood flow

Since the 1950s physicians have noted that plaque collects where blood vessels bend or narrow.[39] Calcification is also found in such areas. Furthermore, when a joint is injured, calcification occurs where blood flow is reduced around scar tissue formation. The precise cause is not known. It can cause acute pain and prevent joint movement due to inflammation and calcification of the tissue, joints, and connective tissue.

Together the conditions described here afflict much of the population of the world. *Most have no cure.* Treatments with anti-inflammatory medicines, steroids, narcotics, and surgery alleviate the symptoms, but usually not the cause.

Given the prevalence of calcification-related diseases among hundreds of millions of patients, it makes sense to ask: Why does educational literature for patients pay virtually no attention to calcium deposits? Perhaps it is because the cause has been unknown until now. Perhaps our specialized medical training systems aren't very good at treating multisystem disorders effectively. Whatever the reasons, the monster that links these ailments often goes unmentioned.

Therefore, it seems high time for someone to explain in plain words how this microscopic malfunction affects us.

CHAPTER THREE

How The "Sand in Our Motor Oil" Plugs Us

Calcification is a pernicious enemy that attacks the tiniest capillaries, the biggest blood vessels, and most organs. It is often accompanied by swelling and clotting that worsens the blockage. Unsurprisingly, at the core of this complex process is the mineral calcium.

The stuff of life…and of death

Chemists know that calcium is a well established part of the periodic table of elements. It was identified in 1808 and is now known to make up roughly three percent of the earth's crust.[1] It is plentiful and widespread.

Calcium is basic to human and animal life. Without it our cells would not function. It is also a critical component of death.

We often think of calcium as a good thing. It is used by our cells to build bones and teeth. Pervasive publicity about calcium supports the idea that it is essential for our well-being. This idea is generally right. As we age we need to watch for calcium loss from our bones because when this happens they get brittle.

Sometimes old and young alike take calcium supplements, although there is contradictory evidence about how much good they do. For example, it has never been fully explained why we need more calcium when reserves in our blood are at normal levels.[2]

With so much emphasis on calcium's advantages, the idea that it is also *bad* for us may come as a surprise.

Biologists have known for decades that too much calcium is a main cause of cell death, just as too little is.[3] For example, too much calcium in nerve cells kills them.[4]

Because of this, the body carefully controls calcium levels to avoid the extremes of overload or starvation.

As we age, we often still have sufficient calcium in us. The problem is that our body doesn't use it in the same way as it does when we are younger.

We might think that harmful calcification would occur when the body has too much calcium, but this is often not the case. One of the mysteries is: *Why does calcification occur when the body's calcium level is normal?* We'll see the answers to that question later.

Calcium takes part in thousands of chemical reactions, including the formation of calcium salts in the human body. We know that these salts are basic ingredients in calcification because they are usually found in autopsied victims who die from related diseases. The main component is a combination of calcium and phosphorous known as calcium phosphate ($CaPO_4$). It is as hard as rock and can scratch some metal.[5] Although it can be manufactured by living organisms, calcium phosphate is remarkably unaffected by antibiotics, other drugs, or radiation that would make our bodies melt.

Pathological calcification is not to be confused with bone and teeth formation—where calcium is used to build the body's framework—or with cell growth that depends on calcium. In our bones and teeth calcium phosphate is used differently to fill in a matrix that supports the frame on which everything else is built. Yet for mysterious reasons calcification strays from these constructive paths to clog our joints, circulation, and organs. One researcher has cut through the scientific jargon by calling it *"sand in our motor oil."*[6]

Start with the tiniest vessels...

A process associated with calcification is sometimes referred to as "microvascular disease." Up to forty billion small blood vessels (capillaries) feed the human body. Most of them are so small that blood cells have to squeeze through them one at a time. Without these capillaries we would die because our cells would not get enough oxygen to survive. Studies have found that capillaries are normally able to expand and contract far more than was known earlier, to control blood flow in the body. So the role of these vessels in our lives is that much greater.[7]

One of the reasons why we feel less energetic as we age is because we are dying slowly as those capillaries harden, swell, and get blocked. At the early stage calcium buildup is preceded by swelling and irritation, combined with buildup of fats. As this clogs blood vessels, it also hardens the passages that deliver blood, nutrients, and oxygen to the body. The corridors get more brittle year after year, and their inability to flex helps to rob us of life-giving nutrients. This also interferes with heart, liver, and other body tissues.

It's an insidious process because we don't sense the onset. Many of us know the later symptoms from experiencing them ourselves or watching others. Everything just gets more difficult. It's tougher to work a full day in top form. We get out of breath more quickly. One day we feel a tightness that isn't supposed to be there. At this point blockages are advanced and body tissue has been compromised. Trouble usually follows.

Exercise and eat right?

Many studies draw links between diet, exercise, and heart disease. If we eat the right types of foods (although as we've seen, there is much argument over what those types are) and exercise the right way, it has been shown that heart disease symptoms are often slowed or may be stopped.[8]

Despite their other undeniable benefits, exercise and eating right do not seem to reverse calcification.[9] As we age, it progresses. Our arteries still get hard, beginning with microvessels, then advancing to the large blood vessels.

In the health and diet aisles of bookstores, thousands of books can be found that touch on heart disease. Yet when it comes to calcium, most of them focus on calcium deficiencies rather than calcification. Remarkably, the indexes of many diet books do not list the terms "pathological calcification" or "calcification."

What's the cause?

Harvard Medical School's Consumer Health information database—one of the more respected sources of medical information for consumers—describes calcification in conditions that are otherwise not usually related. These include illnesses that we've already covered, including heart disease, optical nerve degeneration, erectile dysfunction (difficulty having an erection), gum disease, breast cancer, and spinal cord pain.[10]

Experts at the information database who answer patients' questions state often that there is no known effective way to get rid of calcified areas other than to surgically remove them (a procedure that is too risky in many situations and only a temporary fix in others), or just treat the symptoms.[11]

Experts agree on one other thing: The cause of calcification is murky.[12] In the absence of a known mechanism, it has been relegated to the unexplained.

In this knowledge vacuum tens of billions of dollars are spent annually by patients, insurers, and governments so that doctors can prescribe medicines that let the body stay more or less functional while the underlying condition worsens. This helps to explain why such treatments grow more expensive as time goes by. It is increasingly difficult to conceal painful effects on the body as symptoms get more pronounced.

As we've seen, some researchers suggest that such diseases are triggered by infection,[13] but this is not reflected in explanations that are given to many patients.

Here's a test: Ask your physician what causes calcification. He or she might respond with something like: "Calcification is caused by fatty deposits in the wall of the arteries."[14]

Then ask, "But how do those fatty buildups cause calcification?" Among the standard replies is this bit of techno-speak:

> ...oxygen free radicals create a chemical change (oxidation) in the bad cholesterol. In response, the immune system sends white blood cells to fight this new threat. Unfortunately, the result of the meeting between the white blood cells and the oxidized cholesterol is a fatty plaque that damages the walls of the arteries. These walls gradually narrow, and calcium deposits may collect and harden areas where the walls are inflamed.[15]

In other words, fatty plaque somehow makes calcium salts "collect", then harden.

So, how are these calcium deposits collected? How do they get there? By what mechanism? How does this explain the calcium buildup in non-fatty tissues such as muscles and eyes?

The reply should be that there is no understood way for such fats to collect calcium salts. Nonetheless, a standard response given to patients is that fatty deposits do just that. Since fats and calcium salts come together in artery walls, fatty deposits must trigger calcification.

There are other standard answers aside from these, but they each have the same flaw: There is no proof. No clinical studies have shown that fatty deposits trigger calcification. Yet this assertion is the basis for treatments and low-fat diets that patients are given. In most cases the treatments don't work, or only slow the process instead of reversing it.

Many of us don't know about this calcification dilemma because doctors don't discuss it with us. Nor do consumer medical websites, where patients now get much of their information. A search of the World Wide Web reveals more than one hundred thousand mentions of the term "calcification," with many of those related to calcium buildup in the human body.[16] Yet only a paltry twenty-seven web pages contain the term "cause of calcification."[17] Other such pages discuss the possible cause, but to get at them one has to go into subscriber-based sites often reserved for physicians. Consumers don't normally see these.

Medical journals are full of information about calcification. Billions of dollars are spent researching why calcium deposits end up in the kidneys, gums, and arteries. Medical professionals are acutely aware of the problem, but they and the popular media often do not communicate it to patients because the cause is unknown. Therefore, most of us are in the dark on this vital issue.

Making it worse

Many procedures cause trouble when they are used to cope with the ravages of calcification. During open-heart surgery, heart-lung machines keep patients alive while the heart is shut down for repairs, but the brain is sometimes damaged when capillaries collapse or are blocked, reducing oxygen supply.[18]

Patients who have surgery to restore blood flow often experience re-blockage by inflammation and recalcification, especially at the place where the procedure was performed.[19] Drug company researchers have observed that tubes, known as stents, block less if they contain time-released antibiotics, or are radioactive.[20] Yet these don't stop the process in parts of blood vessels where stents were not inserted.

Kidney and gall stone patients who have their stones pulverized by ultrasound also often experience recurrences. Sometimes the stones come back ferociously.[21]

The infuriating thing is that calcium deposits stare at us each time that we see an X-ray or CT scan. They show up as a white material just as our bones do, only in the wrong places—sometimes in slim lines along the interior of heart valves, or as thorny stones inside our kidneys, or as particles in the brain.

Yet prior to this, a stealthier process generates blockages that often harm or kill us.

The body's own fatal reaction

Calcification is not just accumulation of calcium. Before it can be detected, other symptoms appear. First and foremost is inflammation—swelling that constricts blood vessels just as our throat swells when it is infected. This is the body's way of repairing injuries. The puffiness comes when tiny capillaries expand to let infection-fighting cells pass through their walls to the point of invasion. Swelling in heart disease leads to death when blood flow is interrupted.

A range of fats and fibrous deposits then arrive on the scene as part of the body's attempt to wall off the damage. These biochemical reactions are so numerous and complex that they can confound medical audiences let alone non-medical ones. We cover them in more depth later. What's important is that the interactions lead to development of "soft" and "hard" plaques. Most contain dead cell material that the body can't clear away. Some plaques seem to be part of an attempt to isolate injury to the artery (see Fig. 5).

Finally, there is what many researchers call the "ticking bomb," known as clotting. In an injury, clotting helps to stop bleeding, but in already narrowed arteries it can cause a blockage that leads rapidly to death.[22]

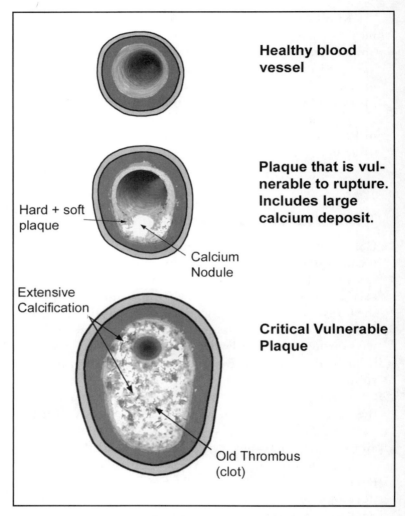

Healthy blood vessel

Plaque that is vulnerable to rupture. Includes large calcium deposit.

Hard + soft plaque

Calcium Nodule

Extensive Calcification

Critical Vulnerable Plaque

Old Thrombus (clot)

Figure 5: The self-destructive process. *Here are snapshots of the decades-long process that leads to blockage of blood vessels by the body's own responses to an invisible enemy. Top: Healthy blood vessel. Center: Plaque buildup with calcium deposits. Bottom: Formula for a heart attack or stroke. The advanced stages of cardiovascular disease. The process can start in childhood. Sometimes it will strike early, but usually it takes decades to accumulate critically. (Illustration courtesy of Dr. Morteza Naghavi, Association for the Eradication of Heart Attack (AEHA) www.vp.org.)*

Researchers have tried for years without success to understand the role of calcification in swelling, plaque formation, and clotting. These are usually found together, and they often kill. At one time it was suggested that calcification may be part of a defensive "walling off" activity to control damage. In that hypothesis, the body uses calcium as a patching material, for example, in cysts that surround infections and cancers. It seems to be applied after other processes, such as swelling, have set the stage by attacking intruders.

However that is a guess. There is no solid evidence that calcium is deliberately put there by the body as a patch. In fact, some researchers argue the opposite to this idea of calcification being used for healing.[23] They say that the body walls off the injured area *including* calcium deposits, by surrounding the deposits with fibrous tissue. This suggests that calcification is the offender and not the cure!

The same researchers also argue that persistent calcification seems to make the defenses go into perpetual overdrive, attempting to wall off an enemy that won't go away.

Until now, exactly why the body does this has been perplexing because it doesn't do it with the calcium in our bones and teeth. If it did, then we'd be dead before we developed fully, as our immune systems attacked the calcium that forms our skeleton. Perhaps the immune system recognizes differences between pathological calcification and calcium that is in our bones. Yet how? Why?

Keep in mind that calcium is the stuff of life. It is used by every cell in the body, not just for bone and tooth manufacturing, but also for growing and dividing. That makes this type of calcium deposit still more mysterious. Why plug arteries that supply life-sustaining blood by depositing calcium that is normally the basis for cell life? It's a classic case of killing the whole to save a part. Oddly, the human body seems to do it incessantly.[24]

Our technology only sees some of it

Much of this blockage is hard to see. The soft tissue buildups, especially inflammation, are virtually invisible on conventional X-rays. They might show up if we take a radioactive dye that lets a machine trace its flow through our arteries to let us see how much they are blocked. But inflammation is still often invisible in such an angiogram.[25] Interpretations of these images are also prone to variation due to the subjective judgments of experts who examine them. The technologies are improving, but they have some way to go before they let us see everything.

We might see more if a physician shoves a catheter through our arteries with a camera attached to it, but such invasive tests are uncomfortable, risky, and expensive. Most of us don't agree to have them done, and doctors don't recommend them, until we have a problem. By then, the condition is seriously advanced.

At a smaller scale, virtually no technology is capable of mapping blockage of the billions of capillaries that make up our microvascular system. The millions of places where blockages begin go undetected. That's one reason why about *half of those who suffer heart attacks show no prior symptoms*.[26] For them, doctors can't predict or see the real situation with regular examination technology.

Some of this problem may soon be solved with sophisticated scanners that let physicians see more soft tissue,[27] but these are very new and haven't yet helped the tens of millions who have blockages now.

In this segment, we've seen that calcification is a dangerous, furtive, inexorable affliction that leads to no end of trouble. It is health enemy number one in many ways. So, what's the cause?

PART II

CATCHING THE CULPRIT

CHAPTER FOUR

The Nano Detectives

Scientists who develop vaccines and test biological products have been perplexed when the cells that they use die routinely after only a few generations. Researchers constantly have to throw out dead cell cultures and start again. This is irritating to companies that develop such products because it is expensive and poses a troubling possibility. The serum might be contaminated with an unknown organism.

Their research depends on growing human or mammalian cells outside the body (*in vitro*). This usually involves fetal bovine serum—often referred to as FBS—which is extracted from calf fetuses and used to help culture cells. The extraction is an ugly process that is opposed by animal rights groups, but researchers argue that vaccines produced this way have saved millions from polio and other diseases.[1] It is a loud dispute.

Contamination of vaccines is a persistent worry. It affects whole populations. For example, polio vaccines were contaminated until about 1963 with a virus known as SV40 that is thought to lead to some cancers.[2]

With such contamination in mind, Dr. E. Olavi Kajander found himself intrigued by the cell-death problem while working in 1985 as a postdoctoral research fellow in the laboratories of Professor Dennis Carson[3] who was then at the Scripps Research Institute in San Diego, California.

This fascination with cell death would eventually lead Kajander to an astounding string of discoveries: A life form so small as to confound standard definitions for being "alive" was inhabiting the human body. It was also triggering calcification that has been tied to many diseases described earlier.

Wrong time, place, and conditions

One project at Prof. Carson's department focused on improving human and mammalian cell culturing. Kajander, who holds a doctorate in biochemistry and is also a medical doctor, used the opportunity to begin exploring why mammalian cells were dying.

Earlier research by scientists at the Coriell Institute for Medical Research—among the largest human cell repositories in the world—suggested that slow-growing microorganisms might exist that could not be detected with standard sterility testing because they did not replicate well under such conditions. Therefore, when Kajander began his quest, it was already suspected that organisms might be present in "sterilized" fetal bovine serum (FBS), but that they did not reveal themselves through routine methods.

Around that same time, entities known as mycoplasmas—organisms without cell walls that are hard to detect—had been discovered that also could not be cultured with standard techniques. They were found to occasionally contaminate cell cultures. It had taken years to find them due to this culturing problem.[4]

Kajander used that history to guess that other contaminants were evading detection. He surmised that researchers were attempting to culture them in *the wrong time frame, with the wrong types of culture media, and under the wrong conditions*. That was when the real detective story began.

To coax these organisms into the open, he began to incubate cell cultures, which were thought to be free of contamination, in a nutrient-rich environment for periods that exceeded normal incubation times. He quickly discovered that something was starting to grow. Its doubling time was extraordinarily long—from three to six days—compared to minutes or hours for most bacteria and viruses. Therefore, it took weeks to develop a "biofilm colony"—a thin slimy layer sometimes excreted by organisms to protect and support themselves—that was big enough to be detected. This supported his hypothesis that an unusually extended incubation time was required. The colony was *not* comprised of mycoplasma that can often contaminate samples. That was important, because some critics would later claim that Kajander had mistaken these entities for mycoplasma.

Looking through a microscope, he saw the first evidence of what would one day be known as *nanobacteria*. It was evidenced by the biofilm that he'd been able to grow.

Where did it come from? Was it present in fetal bovine serum, or were the samples themselves contaminated by accident?

The answer came two years later in 1987 after Kajander returned to Finland to establish his own cell culturing lab at the Biochemistry and Biotechnology Department of the University of Kuopio.

No money but good equipment

Finland may seem like a remote outpost, but many of its universities are known for solid interdisciplinary science. The University of Kuopio, dedicated to medical and biotechnology research, is one such school. A key to Kajander's discovery of nanobacteria was the presence of the newest and best high-tech equipment operated by competent experts in a small university where he had easy access to them. A gamma irradiation facility was available for him to sterilize serum, medium, and equipment. This was to make sure that the contamination was not from the testing equipment or his methods.

After the serum was sterilized with radiation, the mysterious organisms would not grow in it. Then, the organisms were re-injected into the sterile medium and were seen to be growing. This proved that the serum was not contaminated from an outside source.

That may seem like a trivial point, but contamination at such a small scale is a huge problem for researchers. It ruins many experiments. Kajander had to be certain that outside contamination was not the source. Proving this would be central to defending his discovery when it came under scrutiny years later.

The crucial supporters

Kajander was lucky to be at Kuopio for other reasons. Succeeding rectors (Deans) of the University continued to support his work, although the potential for results remained uncertain for years. Moreover, although he himself had virtually no grant money to pay for his research, a professor of anatomy at the university had purchased what was then one of the best light microscopes in the world. Light microscopes are the traditional type of microscope that most of us have seen in high school. They are not as powerful as the newer electron and atomic force microscopes, but the very best ones can see down to the sub-cellular level. This let Kajander see the individual entities in his serum cultures. The vague term "entity" was applied to them because at that time he wasn't certain what they were.

Although the entities were only about a hundred nanometers in size—too small to be seen individually by most light microscopes—their tendency to clump together in their biofilm made them visible under the powerful light microscope that he was using. They were also generating a semi-transparent coating from their biofilm, known as *apatite* (not appetite)—a form of calcium phosphate mineral similar to that found in bones. This made them much larger—about 200 nanometers—and far easier to see.

Oddly, electron microscopes that could see down to a smaller size didn't help at that stage. The rigorous processing steps required to prepare samples to view an as-yet unknown entity under such a microscope resulted in the loss of his hard-to-cut nanobacteria. Their elusive nature confounded sophisticated detection instruments. Instead, it was the best of the "old-fashioned" light microscopes that was used first to crack the case.

In 1990 Kajander asked the Coriell Institute for Medical Research in New Jersey to help him try to identify what these entities were. It had been theorized that perhaps they were mycoplasmas discovered earlier by Coriell Institute scientists. Yet after some investigation by their scientists, assisted by one of Kajander's students, they concluded that they were not mycoplasmas. Unfortunately, the institute also told Kajander that they did not have funding to support further investigation.[5]

Nonetheless, the acknowledgments by Coriell that something was there and that it was not mycoplasma gave Kajander ammunition to argue successfully with his home University of Kuopio in Finland to let him start a small repository to collect cell samples for his experiments. That was a crucial step in the quest that would lead him to find the trigger for calcification.

Patenting natural life?

At that point, he also launched a patent application for isolating and culturing what he was then calling *nanobacterium*. The full name of the genus and species that he'd found in human blood was *Nanobacterium sanguineum,* or "blood nanobacteria." The patent was later accepted in 1992.[6] Its terms were remarkably generous because they covered all methods for detecting nanobacteria and gave Kajander patented jurisdiction over what appeared to be a life form.

Thus, Olavi Kajander became one of the early individuals to patent what seems to be a naturally occurring life form (although as we'll see later there is still a hot discussion over whether this qualifies as a life form according to conventional definitions). Scientists had been patenting genetic modifications to life (such as genetically altered mice) for some time, but until then few if any researchers had acquired a patent on a life form that occurred in nature. It was awarded exclusively to Kajander. Neither his university nor a company were on the application. In an age of corporate and academic competition, this was extraordinary for such a basic discovery.

The patenting of nanobacteria was a profound step in science and law. It foreshadowed what has now become one of the great ethical debates of our time: Who has the right to control life? Because the patent applies to what seems so far as the smallest known form of life, it also suggests that someone might have legal domain over a submicroscopic universe that most researchers know absolutely nothing about.

However, as with other great discoveries—such as the description of DNA years earlier—few experts noticed when the patent was granted. Olavi Kajander slipped quietly into the record books—and into a minefield that would later jeopardize his career.

When he filed for the patent, Kajander also identified antibodies as diagnostic tools to test for nanobacteria's presence. Antibodies are like genetic blood hounds. They sniff out one type of organism and can be used to test for its presence among many others. This was a first step to finding it in samples and in the human body.

The importance of such new diagnostic tools was to prove crucial, because conventional methods for identifying other organisms didn't work with nanobacteria, and would lead other researchers to mis-identify them.

The fetal bovine serum mystery

To find more about what they were and how they grew, Kajander had to find a good medium where a lot of nanobacteria could be cultured. Being strapped for funds, he tried to use the cheapest serum. This led to another discovery. When he compared the cheapest serum with the most expensive, he found more nanobacteria as contaminants in the cheap serum. Therefore, the lower-cost product turned out to be a better source.

That source was fetal bovine serum from the U.K., where fears over Mad Cow Disease (also known as BSE) had rendered the FBS suspect, hence very inexpensive. FBS had been tarred with the same brush as Mad Cow Disease because it came from cow herds in regions where the fatal infection had been identified.

The British serum was full of nanobacteria. This discovery was profoundly significant because it meant that fetal bovine serum from the U.K. was heavily contaminated with nanobacteria. By extension, it suggested that serum used for developing vaccines was also contaminated.

For the next few years Kajander approached manufacturers of fetal bovine serum products and cell culture medium to tell them about the nanobacteria contamination in their serum. The companies agreed that there was a problem with the serum but, according to Kajander, the manufacturers said that they had no customers asking for nanobacteria-free FBS culture media. There was no perceived risk. After all, what diseases did it cause? So from a commercial viewpoint it wasn't interesting or profitable to pay for research to see how the contaminants could be removed.[7]

For Kajander, it was another frustration: The companies whose products were contaminated acknowledged the fact, but they didn't want to act on it by looking for a way to get rid of the contamination.

This had been the same situation that occurred earlier with mycoplasmas. They were discovered in 1950s, but it was not until the 1980s that a demand arose for mycoplasma-free media.[8] Mycoplasma contamination is still a problem today especially with livestock, and eliminating the contaminant is troublesome.[9]

With nanobacteria, history was playing a familiar refrain: experts were unwilling to recognize a new infectious risk, so companies didn't want to fund testing.

The Turkish microbiologist

By 1991, just as Kajander was running out of time and money, one of life's great coincidences transformed his isolated search for the keys to nanobacteria.

One day as he was walking the corridor of his laboratory, the secretary of the department stopped him to ask what she should do with an application from a post-doctoral microbiologist, addressed to the Department of Biology at the University of Kuopio. There was no biology department at the university.

Kajander couldn't believe his luck. A day earlier, he had received a response from the National Institutes of Health in the U.S. telling him that if he wanted to have a grant to explore nanobacteria, then he'd have to find a qualified microbiologist. He took the letter and contacted Dr. Neva Çiftçioglu, who was based in Turkey.

In a telephone interview with her, Kajander sensed her enthusiastic tenacity and hired her forthwith. He hardly had the funds to pay, so the work would have to depend heavily on her own scholarships. In fact, by the time Çiftçioglu arrived, Kajander had temporarily abandoned his experiments on nanobacteria due to financial constraints. Yet, after examining the work that had been done, she was intrigued and continued with the research.

Çiftçioglu would prove to be the missing link in Kajander's quest. She had the microbiological skills that until then had not been applied to basic scientific research on nanobacteria. Like Kajander, she also had experience in medical research, so they shared a deep concern for the mysteries of what made patients sick. With Kajander the biochemist and Çiftçioglu the microbiologist, the combination began to produce results.

The first of many crucial things that she did was to develop special staining methods that would let them see the nanobacteria more easily so that they could be studied. By the end of 1991 she'd succeeded in doing this.

In the years that followed, Çiftçioglu made significant contributions to the original discovery of Kajander's nanobacteria by reducing the time it took to culture them, and by developing unique antibody methods to detect them in living mammals—including humans.

Such methods also led to the eventual founding by Kajander and Çiftçioglu of a company, Nanobac Oy, which offered nanobacteria-related analytical services while research continued at the University.

The accidental contamination

Accidental contamination often ruins experiments, but it also plays a defining role in discovery. Contamination had led researchers to discover penicillin many decades earlier when mold was found to be growing in a petri dish. A similar type of accident catalyzed nanobacteria research.

One day Çiftçioglu confessed to Kajander that she had accidentally contaminated some samples. Kajander was about to scold her because from the start he'd warned her repeatedly against the risk of contamination. However, she was quick to add that it had produced a surprising result. The contamination had shown that nanobacteria had "eaten" the byproducts of the corrupting bacteria as food. It appeared to be a sort of symbiotic process. This discovery let the scientists culture nanobacteria more quickly. It also suggested how the organisms might survive in their environment.

Is "sterile" blood a myth?

The finding of how nanobacteria fed on other organisms shed more light on why they had been missed for so long by other scientists. They required a complex medium in which to replicate relatively quickly. That was present in human urine and blood—media that had been thought by medical science to be normally "sterile," i.e. free of living contaminants.

The idea that human blood was not sterile, but instead might regularly harbor contaminants such as nanobacteria flew in the face of what most medical students had been taught. This arose from the idea that if a contaminant could not be grown from blood by using standard culturing techniques, or seen with conventional methods, then the blood must be sterile.

From the day that medical students enter their training, they are told that blood is a normally sterile environment. If it were not, then we'd probably die because we'd be battling infection in our own blood constantly, causing self-destruction by our immune system as it turned on the body. Yet it now seems that this idea may be flawed.

Kajander's and Çiftçioglu's discovery that nanobacteria survive well in blood constituted part of a string of revelations by many scientists suggesting that blood may not be a normally sterile environment. Pathogens such as *Bartonella* and *Brucella* have also been found to inhabit the bloodstream over extended periods of time.[10] It seems, therefore, that persistent infection in the blood may be more prevalent than was thought. In this respect, the idea

that nanobacteria might roam around the blood for decades is not so special or surprising.

How did so many scientists miss it?

Evidence suggests that the world of nanobacteria may
contain more than just one type of life-like form. It may
contain many new and undescribed types that are vast in
numbers, magnificent in their internal mysteries, and far
more ancient than *Homo sapiens*. Together they may make
up their own submicroscopic universe.

Yet, we have only just begun to discover this universe. Why? The short answer is: We were looking at it,
but we didn't see it.

It is hard to imagine that in an age when most of the
plentiful things on Earth seem to have been discovered,
we'd come across something like this. However, the inability of scientists to recognize plentiful substances has
been repeated throughout contemporary history. A good
example occurred in physics with sub-atomic *neutrinos*
that are now recognized as being among the most abun-
dant substances in the universe. Although their existence
was postulated in mathematics in the 1930s, they could
not be detected for decades because physicists didn't have
the diagnostic tools. Yet neutrinos were passing in the
trillions through every human being, and everything else,
each millisecond of every day.[11]

In the case of nanobacteria, although researchers already had the tools to see them, they didn't recognize
what they were because they lacked the diagnostic methods to isolate and identify their specific components. Clas-
sical methods gave abnormal readings or failed to identify the right characteristics.

Once some of the features of nanobacteria are known,
it becomes clear why they were so hard to find and why
researchers gazed past them daily.

✧ They form a calcium shell that makes them look like a lump of rock instead of something that's alive.

✧ They are hard to isolate with conventional diagnostic tools because they grow at a slow rate and seem to have a unique genetic structure.

✧ They lurk in the twilight zone between life and the chemical processes that spark life.

These features combine to make nanobacteria extraordinarily good at disguising themselves.

Overcoming the barriers to detection

Nanobacteria in their mature calcified form may be seen with a very good conventional light microscope if they are in clusters or biofilm. This does not require a sophisticated electron microscope, which can see far smaller objects. However, it's what's beneath their shell that is important. Preparing samples for a transmission electron microscope often results in loss of nanobacteria because they are so hard to slice into sections for examination. Their small size and special structure also confound conventional preparation methods.

One of Neva Çiftçioglu's tasks was to overcome the detection barriers, especially in the human body. She started by screening kidney stones and dental plaque for nanobacteria. This could only be done after antibodies were developed to do the tests.

Although nanobacteria had been found in fetal bovine serum as early as 1985, it took until the mid-1990s to find them in disease. The delay was due partially to the cost and time to develop "monoclonal antibodies" that are used for finding infections in the human body. The two scientists had to develop the methods themselves, with virtually no outside help.

Also, nanobacteria seem to have a special structure. Their DNA and RNA strands seem unique, and are not yet fully known. The precise gene sequence is hard to detect because chemicals used to strip off the calcium shell may also disrupt their genetic structure. Therefore, regular methods used for gene sequencing had to be modified.

As described earlier, it has also been hard to culture and isolate nanobacteria because they replicate very slowly— over three to six days to produce a daughter cell,[12] instead of just minutes for many bacteria and viruses.

Still one more barrier stopped researchers from finding the culprit. Few dreamed that a self-replicating life form could be as small as 50 to 200 nanometers diameter (see Fig. 6), or that such a tiny thing could generate a calcified coating. Other life-like particles such as viruses can be that small, but they cannot replicate without depending on other life forms to help them, and most do not form calcium coatings.

By together overcoming these barriers to detection, Çiftçioglu and Kajander pried open the doors to the nanobacterial world.

What kills them

Çiftçioglu and Kajander optimized ways of stripping off the apatite coating to get at proteins that were in the nanobacteria. This was essential to determining what they were.

They also discovered that tetracycline and some other chemicals were able to kill the "naked" bacteria once the calcium coating had been removed. In so doing, they found what would later be recognized as crucial components in a treatment for nanobacteria infections: *How to dissolve the protective calcium layer, then kill the underlying organism.*[13]

While these discoveries were unfolding, Kajander and Çiftçioglu sent out the first of many papers that were to be rejected by scientific journals that didn't believe nanobacteria could exist, or demanded expensive and lengthy verification. Such rejections are not unusual. Many renowned discoverers, including Nobel Prize winners, have been rejected by publications early in their careers for similar reasons. It was part of a grueling initiation that Kajander and Çiftçioglu had to get used to.

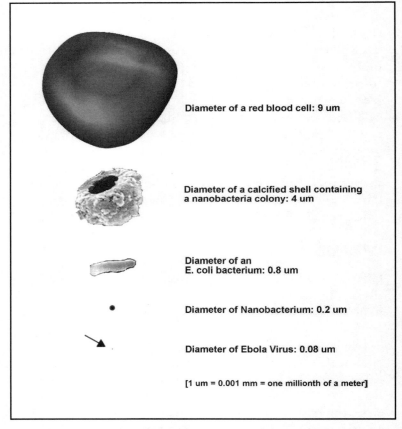

Diameter of a red blood cell: 9 um

Diameter of a calcified shell containing a nanobacteria colony: 4 um

Diameter of an E. coli bacterium: 0.8 um

Diameter of Nanobacterium: 0.2 um

Diameter of Ebola Virus: 0.08 um

[1 um = 0.001 mm = one millionth of a meter]

Figure 6: Rough comparison of average diameters. *A Nanobacterium, dwarfed by a red blood cell, is far smaller than a commonly known bacterium but larger than many viruses. Calcified shell contains many nanobacteria.*

Challenging The Definition
Of Life

Some time ago scientists stunned the world with a claim that "cold fusion" could occur in a test tube. The prospect of limitless cheap energy sparked excitement worldwide, but this dissolved quickly as other researchers reported that they could not duplicate results.[1]

In the biological world, detection and description of the sub-microscopic organism *Nanobacterium sanguineum* were by no means one-off experiments that couldn't be replicated. Instead they began with discovery of the organisms themselves, then progressed to methods for staining them, culturing them, finding them in other media such as vaccines, growing them in lab animals, then isolating them in kidney stones and heart disease. Most—but not all—discoveries were made by the team of scientists in Finland under the leadership of Kajander and Çiftçioglu. Detection of nanobacteria in heart disease was first recorded by one of their collaborators, László Puskás, at the Hungarian Academy of Sciences.[2] His results were later repeated by scientists trained by Kajander at the renowned Mayo Clinic in Rochester and at the Austin Heart Center at the University of Texas.[3] Other scientists at the University of Illinois School of Medicine have detected nanobacteria in kidney disease.[4] Most importantly, as we'll see later, a drug aimed at eradicating them is reversing the signs of heart disease in patients.

Despite this and other work at reputable university institutions, was it still possible that nanobacteria didn't exist, that they were mistaken for something else, and that this was at best an error or at worst a hoax?

Answering that requires some qualifiers:

Due to its tiny size and uncertain structure, *Nanobacterium sanguineum* challenges the very definition of life. Therefore, the skepticism expressed by scientists about its existence is unsurprising. It fits neither the scientific preconception of what is "alive," nor the standard definition of the term "bacterium."

On top of that, it has an "image" problem. It has been confused with everything from chemical processes in ancient earthly rocks, to Martians.

> The idea of the existence of nannobacteria[5] (sic) has been greeted with howls of disbelief by the majority of the biological community, who contend that these minute bodies cannot be bacteria because they are too small to contain the necessary genetic machinery for life.[6]

This excerpt is from a paper by Dr. Robert Folk, the discoverer of geologically-based organisms that he too named nanobacteria. The passage summarizes some of the first shots that were fired at him and other researchers in the fight over whether nanobacteria exist, meet current definitions of being "alive," or are bacteria

The last part of that skeptical question may be right. They are probably not "bacteria" because their structure is different. The question is: Are they too small to be alive?

Folk is credited with being the first to identify such nano scale organisms in geology rock specimens, and it has been said that he did this around 1986, although he didn't publish until many years later.

Enter the Martians

Yet nanobacteria's image problem truly began in 1996. At that time, one of NASA's chief scientists, David McKay, stunned the space exploration community by publishing a paper stating that tiny fossils named nanobacteria had been discovered in a meteorite that apparently came from Mars and had been found in Antarctica.[7] This garnered wide publicity as claims and counterclaims flew over what had been discovered, whether the entities resulted from contamination of samples, and if these were inorganic "artifacts" instead of once-living organisms. The controversy over "Martian life" lent a surreal quality to the nanobacteria discussion. For example, one related article was entitled "The Martians in your kidneys."[8]

Meanwhile, on Earth...

Around the same time geologists led by Philippa Uwins discovered what appeared to be a similar organism in Australia:

> We refer to these features as nano-organisms or nanobes to indicate their significant difference in size to Eubacteria and Archaeae...Our thesis is that nanobes are biological organisms.[9]

The Australian discovery added another feature to the discussion: The presence of RNA and DNA.[10] Was it contamination of samples? Some scientists said yes.

Then in 2002 a team led by Professor Karl Stetter of the University of Regensburg, Germany, discovered nanoscale organisms in volcanic vents in Iceland and named them "nanoarchaeae."[11] The team also announced that they had sequenced the genome.[12]

Thus, DNA was popping up everywhere in nanoscale entities that didn't seem to resemble other types of life: In Australian samples, Icelandic samples, and in *Nanobacterium sanguineum* that triggers disease.

The significance of the nanobacterial phenomena found in geological conditions is not to be underplayed. They may signify existence of the smallest living thing. But so far they have no known scientific link with Kajander's and Çiftçioglu's *Nanobacterium sanguineum* (blood nanobacteria).

Genetic tests are underway at various universities. Until results are published, the link between nanoscale organisms in geological formations and organisms known as *Nanobacterium sanguineum* will be unconfirmed. If a link were to be found, it would be an exciting discovery. Yet right now, early genetic sequences are cryptic and require further testing.

Media confusion between rock and blood nanobacteria started around the later 1990s when information about *Nanobacterium sanguineum* was published in proceedings of conferences where "Martian" nanobacteria were also discussed.

This "guilt by association" wasn't totally bad since it cast new attention on Kajander's and Çiftçioglu's work. Due to the very small size of the Martian nanobacteria, the International Society for Optical Engineering also took an interest in *Nanobacterium sanguineum*. By 1999 a total of nine papers by Kajander and Çiftçioglu about *Nanobacterium sanguineum* had been published in proceedings of the Society's annual meetings. Thus, a tenuous connection with another planet provided an opening to publish.

The connection was a double-edged sword because the Martian meteorite hypothesis had been attacked as nonsense, and the Optical Engineering Society's journal was not regarded as an authoritative source by biological scientists.

Such skepticism was partially dispelled when Kajander's respected mentor at Scripps in California, Professor Dennis Carson, wrote an article in 1998 concluding that nanobacteria were a cause of pathological calcification in humans. That was published in the Proceedings of the National Academy of Sciences.[13]

Still, his acceptance of nanobacteria did not break through the wall of naysayers. Some scientists still claim today that nanobacteria don't exist, or aren't alive. This claim has retarded research into possible nanobacterial infections and treatments for them. Therefore, let's examine the arguments to see if they have merit.

Nanobacteria have been generally defined by their discoverers as nanometer-scale entities that self-replicate and manufacture carbonate apatite structures (calcium phosphate mineral).[14] For a description of some steps in the life cycle of nanobacteria, see Figure 7. However, critics claim:

1. Nanobacteria don't exist.

Here is a summary of the conflicting possibilities put forward by supporters and opponents:

✧ Possibility A: Various organisms of nanometer size (billionths of a meter) have been found by scientists looking at thousands of samples from meteors, volcanoes, geological core samples, vaccines, and blood taken from locations around the world. Some have had their gene sequences mapped. They seem to be new forms of life, although they are not yet shown to be related.

✧ Possibility B: Although scientists from institutions around the world have found, cultured, and sometimes gene sequenced nanobacteria, all of these findings resulted from experiments that were contaminated. Or, they found non-living entities that attract DNA and can self-replicate without being alive.

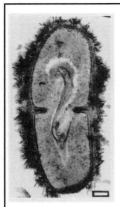

The birth of an organism? — According to its discoverers this is a replicating nanobacterium 250 billionths of a meter thick. Millions would fit onto the head of a pin. Note the "hairy" apatite layer around the exterior. This is solidifying calcium phosphate. (Bar in picture = 100 nm.)

A colony of nanobacteria hanging together with biofilm. It takes weeks or months for one nanobacterium to replicate enough times to produce such a colony. (Bar = 1 μm.)

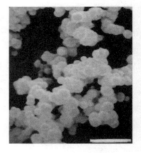

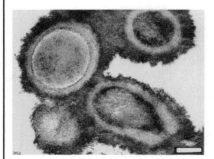

A group of nanobacteria beginning to congregate and form a calcified shell that will contain the colony [picture taken after 3 months culturing period] (Bar = 200 nm)

Figure 7: Various lifecycle stages of nanobacteria.
Photos are copyright (1998) National Academy of Sciences, U.S.A.[15]

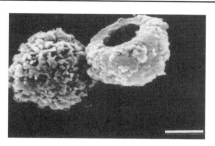

Scientists have been staring at these igloo-like structures for decades. They often are found at the centers of kidney stones. The structures shown here were grown outside the human body without serum. This simulates the growth conditions in the human body when the nano-bacteria have been cut off from nutrients by the body's defensive response. Under those conditions nanobacteria increase biofilm pro-duction and form these hardening shells. Nanobacteria semi-hiber-nate in the protection of these structures, but still produce buds. The flat side of the igloo above, where the hole is located, marks where the shells were attached to the petri dish. (Bars = 1 μm.)

The beginning of a long, deadly war. Nanobacteria attacking healthy cells. By infiltrating the cells, nano-bacteria get the energy and resources to replicate. But they also trigger an immune response in the body that results in inflammation, clotting, and dangerous deposits.

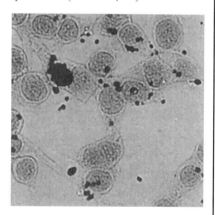

Figure 7 (continued).

✧ Possibility C: It's all a hoax. The scientist who
   purported to make the discovery used fraudulent claims to pull the wool over the eyes of
   many reputable institutions, although they
   replicated his results in their own experiments
   many times.

2. Something is there (but it's not bacteria and it's not alive).

Given the breadth of evidence it seems certain that they
have found *something* (see Fig. 7). It is further possible
that these "somethings" are each dramatically different
and that blood nanobacteria and geological "nanobacteria"
are unrelated. Advanced DNA sequencing techniques should
soon give us the answers to that.

The "something" found by Kajander and Çiftçioglu
contains fragments of DNA and RNA that are associated
with initiation of life processes. It also seems clear that
they have found that entity in the human body and that
it exhibits the characteristics of being infectious.

Critics claim that a self-replicating crystalline structure—in other words a rock that grows chemically—could
exhibit or cause each of these characteristics. It could also
accidentally contain DNA captured from living material.
Yet the crystals themselves are not alive.[16]

Defenders have shot back that this is like trying to fit
a round peg into a square hole: Instead of establishing a
new category in which to put a newly discovered organism, critics try to stuff it into a conventional box.

Other critics bring up the "C" word: Contamination
of samples. It is thought that contamination with DNA
from other sources is what all these scientists are finding.
Contamination is nothing new, and it is a big problem at
this scale. However, it can be misused as a convenient
explanation when die-hard opponents run out of other

arguments. So without other proof that contamination occurred it has to be taken with a grain of salt.

Still other scientists argue that the smallest possible size for a free living, DNA-based organism is a diameter in the size range of 200 to 250 nanometers.[17] Anything smaller, they argue, cannot contain the types of DNA and other materials required for something to be "alive" by commonly accepted definitions. Nanobacteria have been identified in the 50-300 nanometer range, putting them near or below that minimum size.

Yet Kajander himself has pointed out that some of the smaller items may not be complete nanobacteria, but rather "buds," or fragments, from larger mature nanobacteria.[18] He is one of the first to emphasize that these smaller fragments may not themselves be "alive" in the conventionally accepted sense. He adds that nanobacteria may force us to redefine what is "alive," due to their special structure.

Normally people think that a living entity is a cell—that it is surrounded by a membrane and that it is a closed compartment. Now we face a possibility that nanobacteria may consist of elementary units that on their own are so very small that they may have to come together to make a living organism.[19] Furthermore, before they self-assemble into larger units, these smaller units may rely on a host organism to survive.[20]

Kajander also cites a new argument by some scientists that the smallest living thing is a single gene—something far smaller than a cell—and that genes come together to form larger living entities.[21] That, he says, also challenges the definition of living organisms.

Another problem, as mentioned earlier, is the "bacteria" part of the name. The discoverers point out somewhat regretfully that this leads scientists to try to compare the organisms with well-known types of bacteria such as *E.coli* (bacteria found in the intestines) that are much larger and have a different genetic structure.[22] Yet DNA tests suggest that nanobacteria are a different type of organism because they do not respond to the standard form of DNA testing.

When does a primordial thing containing complex chemicals and genes—and exhibiting life-like behavior—become alive? Is it possible that nanobacteria have some characteristics of life, but other characteristics of non-life that somehow put them in a category of their own? Viruses and prions have their own categories. It is still debated as to whether they are alive or not. Why should the same ambivalence not be accepted for nanobacteria?

The ugly parts

The hard discussion began in 1999 when the journal *Nature* published an article reporting that a group of academics in Finland had accused nanobacteria discoverer Olavi Kajander of unethically overstating results of his research. No one was more surprised than Kajander, who first read about it from that journal. The accusation was coming from someone who, according to Kajander, had done no laboratory research of his own on the organism. Still, one journalist went after the story this way:

> A Finnish scientist has formally asked the University of Kuopio to investigate the work of one of its senior researchers, who, he says, is making misleading but widely publicized claims to have discovered a new form of life, known as nanobacteria.
>
> Over the past few years, a group of Finnish scientists have expressed concern that Olavi Kajander has failed to produce the necessary biochemical evidence to prove that the particles he claims to be nanobacteria are in fact alive. Kajander says that he has shown this, and he has supporters of his own, including some prominent researchers at the US space agency NASA.[23]

It was especially surprising because the patent for a nanobacterium, along with methods for detecting and culturing it had been granted to Kajander many years earlier. [24]

After a formal investigation, the University of Kuopio's Ethics Committee, where the complaint was filed, concluded in 2000 that:

> Issakainen's written and oral reasoning implies interpretative opinions on the results of Kajander's research and their documentation. In the view of the Research Ethics Committee this is a matter of scientific dispute and not of misconduct or fraud in science.

> The Rector has examined the documents and the data presented and has concluded that the request for investigation by Jouni Issakainen, [M.Sc.], warrants no further actions by the Rector.

> The complaint by Jouni Issakainen...against Docent [full Professor], research director Olavi Kajander, Ph.D. is herewith rejected. [25]

So, the complaint was thrown out as unfounded; not once but twice, when one of the central scientific ethics committees of Finland also rejected it. [26]

Unfortunately, the news of Kajander's vindication couldn't reverse the damaging delay that resulted to some of his work. His exoneration also went unreported in the journal *Nature*, where the original story had run. This episode exemplifies how just the news of an accusation can set back research, especially if science media don't cover the outcome of an official investigation after its beginnings have already been reported.

The controversy escalated when an American researcher John O. Cisar, using a grant from the U.S. National Institutes of Health, wrote a paper with other scientists explaining that they had only partially replicated Kajander's results. They were able to culture the entities and take electron microscope photographs of them, but were unable to identify that they contained DNA unique to that life form. The Cisar team concluded that:

> ...these data do not provide plausible support for the existence of a previously undiscovered bacterial genus. Instead, we provide evidence that biomineralization previously attributed to nanobacteria may be initiated by nonliving macromolecules and transferred on "subculture" by self-propagating microcrystalline apatite.[27]

In other words, although the researchers reported that they were able to culture them and photograph them, these entities could not be bacteria and were not alive because the experiment hadn't managed to characterize them.

FDA advisory group discounts nanobacteria

On the basis of an interpretation of that finding, an arm of the U.S. Food and Drug Administration (FDA) concluded that nanobacteria don't exist, therefore are not potential contaminants in vaccines.

Here is how their conclusion seems to have been reached:

In November 2002, as part of their regular quarterly meeting, officials from the FDA's Vaccines and Related Biological Products Advisory Committee[28] discussed a new potential contaminant that allegedly had been found in bovine and human serum used for products such as children's injectable polio vaccines and Human Immune Globulin. The meeting participants listened as Dr. Dennis Kopecko, chief of one of the FDA laboratories, summarized the work of Kajander and his colleagues, who had suggested that such contamination may play a role in heart disease and kidney stones that are related to deposition of calcium in the human body.[29]

Kopecko explained that none of this contamination was likely to have occurred, because according to him, Dr. Kajander had misinterpreted the data.[30] The gene sequence found in tests by a team that Kopecko participated in resembled that of another type of bacteria, *Phyllobacterium*.[31] According to him, there was—and still is—no credible molecular evidence to support the existence of nanobacteria.[32]

Furthermore, he believed that the other structures seen by his group and Kajander's were non-living hydroxyapatite crystals, not nanobacteria. Therefore, identification by Kajander of nanobacteria looked to Kopecko like a mistake.

The possibility of such contamination was subsequently dismissed by the committee for the time being.[33]

In so doing, the committee depended heavily on the experiment and paper by John O. Cisar, Kopecko and others,[34] that according to Kajander and Çiftçioglu used incomplete methods for characterizing the organisms. The Cisar team, they say, reached the right results by culturing the entities, but did not use commercially available controlled culturing techniques and verifying methods to avoid contamination.[35] Kajander also says that Cisar had found only weak signs of DNA because nanobacteria have a special DNA strand that does not respond well to the type of detection methods used by Cisar.[36] The DNA detection problem is especially relevant because it suggests again that nanobacteria have a unique DNA structure, different from other known organisms.

Such issues had been discussed with the FDA earlier. Prior to the committee's regular session, a meeting had occurred between Kopecko's group and Kajander and Çiftçioglu, in which possible reasons for the Cisar team findings were discussed. What was actually said at that meeting is disputed among attendees. Among the many contentious points, most focus on methods and interpretations used by each side.

Both teams claim that the other's samples were contaminated.[37] The Cisar team found *Phyllobacterium* in their own tests, and deduced from this that Kajander's and Çiftçioglu's tests were also contaminated with the bacterium. Wrong, say Çiftçioglu and Kajander.

Nanobacteria resemble *Phyllobacterium* in some ways, but they can be differentiated in structure, growth requirements, biochemistry, and antigen patterns, which are accepted methods for telling organisms apart.

Some of this comes back to DNA. Kopecko says that there is none evident to support nanobacteria. Kajander counters that while the DNA of nanobacteria has not been fully characterized so far, careful methods are required to isolate the type of DNA that sets it apart from organisms such as *Phyllobacterium*. He says that the Cisar tests failed "because he did not use the best techniques and got all tests contaminated."[38]

Thus, everybody seems to agree on one thing: more DNA testing is required.

In the absence of complete DNA identification then, what are the telling factors that set nanobacteria apart?

Kajander and his colleagues list many features that distinguish them from other organisms. Among these are differing reactions to antibiotics, disinfectants, and radiation (see Fig. 8). The researchers argue that many such features could not be exhibited by non-living crystals.

In view of such arguments, it seems odd that prior to discounting evidence that nanobacteria are a potential problem in vaccines the committee did not suggest that critics and proponents do such specialized experiments under independent monitoring, and also try and distinguish other characteristics of nanobacteria. This is especially perplexing when so many reputable institutions have published findings of nanobacteria in disease. Scientists at the University of Illinois found nanobacteria in kidney and brain disease, as we'll discuss later. Then in 2002 Mayo Clinic researchers reported that they were able to identify nanobacteria in human arterial plaque.[39] This confirmed unpublished results that had been produced earlier by Hungarian Academy of Sciences researcher Dr. László Puskás.[40] On top of that, in 2003, researchers from the Panum Institute, University of Copenhagen, and the University of Ulm, Germany, said they completed experiments indicating that the apatite formation observed with nanobacteria is generated by a process normally only seen in living organisms.[41]

Such findings tend to reinforce a troubling question: What if Çiftçioglu and Kajander are *right* about vaccine contamination? Might the FDA be looking back some day

Property	*Nanobacterium sanguineum*	Viral particles	Prion particles	Bacteria
Size [nm]	50 - 300	20 - 250	<250	>250
Self-replicating	yes	no	no	yes
Resistance to gamma-irradiation [Mrad]	~2.5	< 2.5	> 2.5	<0.1->6.0
Resist boiling	yes	no	yes	no
Resist disinfectants	yes	some	yes	no
Resist antibiotics	most all	yes	yes	resistant to some
Cause inflammation	yes	yes	no	yes
Cause host cell death	yes	yes	specific	some
Cause pathologic calcification	yes	a few	no	a few
Form biofilms	yes	no	no	yes
Found in atherosclerotic plaque	yes	some	no	a few

Figure 8: How to tell *Nanobacterium sanguineum*. *Here are a few defining characteristics of "blood nanobacteria" that, according to their discoverers, make them special. This table shows how they are similar to, and different from, other types of pathogens.[42]*

wondering why this was not analyzed further when it was brought to their attention?

Is it possible that something slipped past the stringent filtering and sterilization techniques used to protect vaccines against just such contamination? Although it is a rare occurrence, it wouldn't be unprecedented. Some viruses eluded capture in blood serum for many years.[43]

Despite such concerns, Kajander and Çiftçioglu emphasize that there is no reason to stop taking vaccinations. They say that nanobacteria are slow growing and less immediately dangerous compared to the effects of diseases that vaccines prevent.

Meanwhile, other scientists had still been producing studies claiming that nanobacteria couldn't be found, then concluding that they might not exist. In 2003 a group in France produced one such study. A telling element was that they admitted that they were unable to generate biofilm in their samples, although various other researchers have reported being able to do so.[44] Neither did they mention the 2002 Mayo results in their references. Nor, according to Çiftçioglu, did they consult with her team on methodologies for the tests.[45]

It started with the kidneys...

In the related controversy over whether calcification derives from nanobacteria, some of the more intriguing evidence lies not in the petri dish but in the kidneys.

About one in ten persons develops kidney stones in their lifetime. Those who live and work with sufferers are also affected because kidney stones cause the most excruciating distress. When the stones get stuck in the urinary tract or begin to move along it, they can instantly debilitate the strongest individual. Men who have these attacks sometimes say that they know how painful it must be to give birth. Many women say that passing a kidney stone feels far worse. Calcium deposits that make up most of these stones form a jagged series of outcroppings, known as spicules, around a solid core. When they move down the urinary tract, these spurs scrape the nerves raw and also cause the stone to stick in the passageway.

The prevalence of kidney stones among Americans and Europeans has been increasing for the past twenty years, but no one knows why. The exact cause of most stones is also still unknown, although it has been linked to diet, lifestyle, and heredity.[46] Once someone gets such stones, they are prone to recurrences. This is especially true with patients who have stones surgically removed or pulverized by shock wave therapy.[47]

The most common stone is made of calcium compounds. A rarer stone, known as a struvite, is caused by another type of well known infection in the urinary tract,[48] but this is not the case with most stones. Thus, calcification plays a major part in most stone formation.

One conventional explanation for how the most common stones form goes something like this: For unknown reasons, crystals of calcium stick to the insides of the kidneys. Normally these are excreted in urine, but in some cases they are not. These calcium crystals congregate to form stones.[49]

The igloo

Researchers have noticed for decades that as kidney stones form, the crystalline structures that are near their core have a hollow "igloo" shape to them.[50] The intriguing thing is that crystalline processes are not normally known to chemically manufacture such structures without the presence of living organisms.

In 1996, Neva Çiftçioglu's brother Vefa Çiftçioglu, a Turkish dentist who had been researching nanobacteria in periodontal disease, urged her to investigate the link between nanobacteria and kidney stones. He himself had developed stones, although there was no history of them in the family. He suspected that he had been infected.

When Neva Çiftçioglu began examining dissected stones through an electron microscope, she was astonished to find that the igloo-like structures that she'd seen growing some years ago in a petri dish of cultured nanobacteria (see Fig. 7) were the same ones at the heart of the kidney stones. On top of that, most of these "cores" tested positive for nanobacteria.

By 1998 Çiftçioglu and Kajander had reported their findings in the Proceedings of the National Academy of Sciences.[51] They theorized that nanobacteria were acting as "nidi" (centers) in kidney stone formation.

Just prior to that, researchers from the University of Illinois, Drs. Thomas Hjelle and Marcia Miller-Hjelle had read about nanobacteria and contacted Dr. Olavi Kajander to suggest collaboration on investigating Polycystic Kidney Disease (PKD). This hereditary disease, affecting more than 12 million victims worldwide, results in multiple cysts that cause the kidneys to swell and eventually stop working. At that stage dialysis and transplants are the only treatment.[52]

As with heart disease, microbes were suspected of triggering PKD, but no one was able to isolate them. The evidence pointing to an infection was even stronger than in heart disease, because toxins from bacteria had often been identified in the fluid that came from such cysts.[53]

In their tests the Hjelles extracted fluid from the cysts and checked for nanobacterial antibodies and antigens. Nanobacterial antigens were found in 75 percent of the cases, and the nanobacteria themselves were cultured from many of the specimens.[54]

This work by University of Illinois and University of Edinburgh experts was crucial, because it took the medical study of nanobacteria into some of the most respected medical institutions. Once such institutions were involved it was more difficult for critics to claim that findings were restricted to one or two researchers.

The case of Randall's Plaques

Earlier in 1998 Çiftçioglu, Kajander, and the Hjelles also met with University of Chicago Professor Fredric Coe, founder of Litho-link, a testing and disease management service for kidney stone patients. Coe is a leading kidney stone researcher and practitioner, who is noted for his success in reducing kidney stone recurrence in patients.

According to Kajander and Çiftçioglu, when they showed him photographs of the igloo-like structures, Coe went to his library and brought back a journal article published decades earlier by Dr. Alexander Randall, a pioneering kidney researcher known for identifying formations named "Randall's Plaques." The article described those same structures in the plaques.

Çiftçioglu maintains that this special igloo may be central to the argument about whether nanobacteria exist or are alive. She says that the detection and culturing of nanobacteria from the core of such structures undermines the argument that a non-living crystalline process produces such structures.

Coe began to examine the formation of kidney stone cores as part of a multimillion-dollar NIH-funded study that had gone on for some years.[55] By 2003, as part of that work, he and other researchers produced evidence that the smallest pieces of plaque in kidneys were composed of calcium phosphate.[56] This was the same material that the Hjelles had found in the igloo-like structures. Was there a link? Coe didn't speculate, nor did he associate the work with that of the Hjelles, but it was clear from his research that some of the dominant theories about kidney stone formation were being refuted.

Prof. Coe wasn't the only one to go after such formations. In 2002, the Mayo Clinic stepped up an investigation into nanobacteria in kidney stones, having identified them in their own independent analysis earlier.[57]

The false positive

It was also during the kidney investigations that Kajander, Çiftçioglu, and the Hjelles came across a remarkable co-incidence that may help to solve one of the great myster-ies of heart disease.

We saw in Chapter 1 that many bacteria and viruses have been identified in arterial plaque that typifies heart disease. One of those is *Chlamydia pneumoniae*. To de-tect this, a commonly applied commercial test is used. For years the test has been employed to find evidence of *Chlamydia* in plaques. However, there has also been a big problem. Once scientists found the indicator, they often could not culture the *Chlamydia*. Many studies note this contradiction.

While looking for nanobacteria in kidney stones, the University of Illinois team came up with an astounding finding: Nanobacteria give off a "false positive" for *Chlamy-dia* when the commercial test is used.[58] The same cross-reactivity was found for a bacterium known as *Bartonella*, which has also been detected in heart disease. Thus, for years scientists may have been getting false positives gen-erated by nanobacteria, when they thought that they were detecting *Chlamydia* and *Bartonella*. This explains why sometimes they couldn't culture *Chlamydia* and *Bartonella*. In those cases, they just weren't there. This does not mean that *Chlamydia* and *Bartonella* don't play a role in kidney or heart disease. Instead it suggests that some-thing precedes their presence.

A trigger, but not the whole story

The experience with nanobacteria in kidney stones and Polycystic Kidney Disease resembles patterns found in other calcific diseases. According to their discoverers, nanobacteria are not the total story, but instead seem to be ongoing triggers that allow the diseases to take hold. Once the diseases get a lock on the body, other processes come into play. These may repeatedly accelerate, then seem to disappear, but they ultimately cause the symptoms to snowball.

This at once explains why nanobacteria are so hard to get at—because they are walled off by cyst-like formation processes—and why getting rid of nanobacteria doesn't immediately fix damage caused by accompanying diseases—because the damage may be complex and well advanced.

That becomes a crucial factor later when we look at the treatment that has been developed, then respond to the question "*Has heart disease been cured?*"

What is life?

By 2003, so many defective methods had been used to try and isolate *Nanobacterium sanguineum* that Kajander, with his researcher colleague and wife Katja Aho as lead author, wrote the *Journal of Clinical Microbiology* to outline the pitfalls, so that researchers might avoid wrongly concluding that nanobacteria didn't exist or did not exhibit life-like properties.[59] Furthermore, they explained that nanobacteria *are* alive because, among other things;

- ✧ The formation of a biofilm from cultured nanobacteria shows that they self-replicate as living cells do.

- ✧ Heavy doses of gamma radiation eliminate the biofilm. This strongly suggests that the organisms have been killed. To be killed, they have to be alive in the first place.

- ✧ They are killed with a broad spectrum antibiotic.[60]

See Fig. 8 for properties of *Nanobacterium sanguineum* in relation to other pathogens.

When we see how such properties set nanobacteria apart from other pathogens, it becomes apparent that a big problem with a nanobacterium is its *name*. Scientists may come to understand it as something altogether different from conventional bacteria.

Nonetheless, after all is said and done, the question arising from these debates is:

So what?

Something doesn't have to be "alive" in the conventional sense to cause trouble in the body. For example, debates go on today over whether viruses are "alive." Some researchers argue that they cannot replicate on their own, therefore they lack one of the conditions to be classified as living organisms.[6] Yet they contain RNA and DNA, and they cause no end of harm. Likewise, tiny protein particles known as prions, some of which are known to cause Mad Cow Disease (also known as BSE), are not considered to be alive, yet they too cause much trouble and can kill.

Does it matter whether nanobacteria are seen as alive or not in the conventional sense? To thousands of researchers it matters very much, because this is the stuff of Nobel prizes—defining the limits of life, or finding a new form of life that has deep implications for the human organism. Yet to patients, it does not matter.

What truly matters

For millions of disease sufferers who have run out of options and need new solutions right now, here is what truly matters. First and foremost, nanobacteria don't care what we call them—they still seem to harm and kill us in great numbers. Also, according to the discoverers:

✧ Particles of apatite found in the blood are toxic. They do not have to be alive to kill a human. The most important thing is to get rid of them.

✧ Entities named *Nanobacterium sanguineum* are found in the apatite that permeates arterial plaque, kidney stones, and other disease sites. Patients with these diseases test positive for the pathogen.

✧ Above everything else, a special combination of chemicals and drugs kills the nanobacteria and, as we'll see later, reverses associated symptoms in cardiovascular disease.

Alive or dead, organisms or not, it's not so much what they *are* as what they *do*. Whatever they do seems to harm us.

CHAPTER SIX

Seeds Of Destruction?

By 2002 scientists from high profile medical research institutes were hot on the trail of nanobacteria. Here is a mouthful of terminology written by some of them. It may yet confirm a great discovery:

> Positive immunological staining for nanobacteria was... heterogeneously distributed both in areas showing positive and negative staining for calcium phosphate. ...immunohistochemical and anatomical characteristics provide evidence of nanometer-scale structures in calcified human cardiovascular tissue. These structures are similar to nanobacteria described and isolated from human kidney stones and geological specimens. These observations fulfill one criterion for Koch's postulate to suggest that a calcifying "nanobe" could participate in calcification of vascular tissue.[1]

In plain English it means that researchers from the Mayo Clinic and University of Texas had confirmed what Hungarian researcher Dr. László Puskás had already discovered. Entities known as nanobacteria are in the plaque associated with coronary heart disease.

Perhaps because such a claim was so significant, it took the academic reputation of American universities to convince a medical journal to publish something that no journals would publish years earlier.

Moreover, a few years prior to the Mayo Clinic announcement, a practitioner by the name of Dr. Gary Mezo, based in Tampa Florida, had invented and started to administer a treatment that targeted nanobacteria in heart disease. The encouraging results from his early patients gave further support to the Mayo Clinic and University of Texas research findings. We'll get to Dr. Mezo's pivotal role in upcoming chapters. We mention him now because much of the theorizing that is described here regarding the role of nanobacteria in atherosclerosis comes from him as well as the others mentioned in this chapter. Yet before we cover the treatment that he developed, we first have to explain how the related infectious process seems to work.

Why do we calcify under normal conditions?

We've seen that there is nothing new about finding bacteria or viruses in heart disease because many such infections have already been identified. The new thing is that a special organism has been seen to grow a calcium shell, just like the calcification found in arterial plaques.

Earlier research has found that calcification accumulates in arteries at a steady rate, making it unnoticeable in its early stages, but potentially fatal as the mass grows in later years.[2] This apparent doubling of calcium deposits every few years may explain why so many patients with no apparent signs of heart disease die suddenly. In a young adult the doubling of a tiny growth might go unnoticed for decades. Yet in its advanced stages the resulting blockage of blood vessels may go from partial to total, causing a "sudden" crisis, especially when combined with the equally dangerous threats of swelling and clotting.

According to some researchers, nanobacteria are the only known pathogens to grow a calcified shell in conditions where calcium is not plentiful and acidity is neutral.[3] Kajander and his colleagues found that nanobacteria suck calcium out of their surroundings, then combine it with other chemicals and compounds (some of which are known commonly as cholesterol or lipids) to secrete a slime known as biofilm.[4] Then Çiftçioglu later found that this solidifies into an armor of calcium mineral (known as hydroxyl apatite). The capacity to generate such a shell under these conditions seems unique to nanobacteria.

This then answers the critical question that we asked in an earlier chapter about the role of calcium:

Why does harmful calcification occur when calcium levels in the body are normal?

Some other bacteria can generate another form of calcification known as calcium carbonate,[5] but none are known to manufacture "apatite" or calcium phosphate under such conditions.[6]

Once nanobacteria are encased in their shell, they go into a semi-dormant state. On casual examination they look like microscopic pebbles (see Fig. 7). The shell is hard to strip off. It resists high heat, radiation, and drugs. A scientist can examine the shell under an electron microscope, yet without training still not see the nanobacteria that are in it. This has led some to dismiss it as a calcium "artifact."

Why nanobacteria are so dangerous

According to the researchers who discovered them, nanobacteria:

- ✧ Maim and kill healthy cells
- ✧ Trigger persistent swelling and clotting
- ✧ Suck calcium and cholesterol from the blood to form deposits that clog us
- ✧ Cause the body to wall them off with fibrous-fatty plaques that begin to block blood vessels

✧ Form part of a complex of soft plaque that accumulates year by year, causing health problems.

To demonstrate some of these capabilities, researchers explain that when nanobacteria are injected into a previously uninfected animal, they concentrate in the kidney cells. Kidney stones then form, like stalactites hanging from the roof of a cave.[7] This is one of the ways that nanobacteria make us sick.

The disease-triggering process

Olavi Kajander and Neva Çiftçioglu, who discovered nanobacteria and how to kill it, and Gary Mezo, who discovered a treatment that gets rid of it in human subjects, summarize the state of their emerging theories about the disease-triggering process this way, as paraphrased by the authors. [*It must be emphasized here, as indicated by Dr. Benedict Maniscalco in the Foreword to this book, that much research remains to be done prior to every part of these theories being definitively established.*[8]]

It is known that nanobacteria emit a slime-like calcium and fat-laden biofilm.[9] This biofilm acts as a type of "Trojan Horse," and makes them attractive to large healthy cells. Those cells suck the biofilm containing nanobacteria through their protective external membranes into their own vulnerable interiors.

Absorbing food through its membrane is a regular function for a cell. That's how it eats. Unfortunately, many pathogens have learned how to trick cells into absorbing them. The results of this Trojan Horse-like infiltration are often fatal. The nanobacteria consume the internal parts of infected cells to get the resources and energy to produce a calcium shell that protects them when the body's immune system tries to wall off the area of nanobacterial infection.

In response to being cut off from their nutritional supply—blood—the nanobacteria form their shell and become semi-dormant. In this armor, they are still able to multiply and generate more calcium that adds to their covering, and also continue to stimulate the immune response. As such the progression of disease may alternatively accelerate or diminish, but never stops.

Ironically, our own defensive mechanisms cripple us when they try to kill nanobacteria. In reaction to the biofilm emitted by the nanobacteria, and also in response to the nanobacterial calcium deposits, our immune systems trigger a process that surrounds them with soft fibrotic tissue. The mechanism appears to operate like a cyst forming around an infection. This soft tissue is found in most arterial blockage. The accumulation of tissue, calcification, and inflammation is chronic and life-long. Ultimately, it leads to coronary artery disease when the processes block first small, then large, passageways. (For further expansion of this concept see Appendix entitled "How Nanobacteria May Trigger The Atherosclerotic Process.")[10]

Cows don't have to be mad to be infectious

What is the source of nanobacteria, and is it possible to stop them before they enter the human body? The list of possible origins is long and under-investigated. Everything from Martian meteorites to underground or underwater repositories has been suggested. Many people eat red meat, and because calcium-encased nanobacteria may not be killed by cooking they might enter us that way. Urine from infected animals and humans has high nanobacteria levels and may contaminate drinking water sources. One study suggests that they may be in some water supplies.[11] Due to their size and resilience, conventional purification may not protect us from them. Studies have not yet been published on the presence of nanobacteria in plants, so it is not certain that we are infected when we

eat them. The presence of nanobacteria in livestock suggests that they may come from some environmental source.[12]
So, nanobacteria may be distributed throughout our environment, but whether we develop disease from that
depends on our surroundings, how many contaminated
vectors we are exposed to, and our genetic abilities to
fight infection.

One area is known where it may be possible to stop
the contamination. That is fetal bovine serum, the same
medium that Olavi Kajander used to find nanobacteria in
the 1980s.

> How are humans exposed to nanobacteria? Cows seem
> to be hosts to nanobacteria and biopharmaceutical
> products from cell culture (fetal bovine serum used as
> a supplement) are occasionally contaminated with
> nanobacteria. Such a contamination has been recently
> reported in viral vaccines. About 15% of human serum
> samples from healthy blood donors contain anti-
> nanobacteria antibodies and nanobacteria can be occa-
> sionally found and cultured from serum…As the first
> phase we screened presence of nanobacteria markers
> in 7 commercial gamma globulin products. We found
> that nanobacteria antigen was culturable in 2 out of 7
> preparations studied.[13]

Is such contamination a problem?[14] Does it seem to
be life threatening? Is it possible to stop nanobacteria by
stopping the use of fetal bovine serum? Is there some link
with beef-related diseases? No one knows the answers,
because the investigations have not been done yet.

Nonetheless, as more researchers begin to find
nanoscale organisms in human or serum samples, and
with discovery of why mammalian cells die in fetal bovine
serum in many laboratories, it seems prudent to start
looking for sources of entry into the human body.

Right now the more compelling issue is: How do we
get rid of the bad calcification that's already in us and
that poses a clear and present threat?

PART III

TREATMENT

CHAPTER SEVEN

The Entrepreneurial Practitioner

> When you look at the thought that there is possibly a
> way to approach a (coronary) plaque, break it down,
> remove the offending pathogen, and eliminate that
> plaque, then that's...astounding.[1]
>
> > Benedict S. Maniscalco, M.D., F.A.C.C., commenting
> > on a nanobiotic treatment developed
> > by Dr. Gary Mezo

Thousands of heart disease patients might be dead today or at least seriously incapacitated if it were not for the compassionate entrepreneurialism of Dr. Gary Mezo, who found a way through the red tape.

While debates raged over whether nanobacteria were alive, many physicians were noticing that heart patients who were being treated with Mezo's prescription drug were doing something unusual. They were not dying. On top of that, they were improving.

Mezo came onto the nanobacteria scene years after Kajander and Çiftçioglu made their first discoveries. Yet there is no doubt that his contribution was monumental. Besides his own earlier discovery of a heart disease treatment, he also found a way to bring benefits to patients who had no other hope. By so doing he leapfrogged over years of regulatory roadblocks into the realm of treating human patients. This singular achievement succeeded partially because *many heart patients had exhausted their options and faced imminent death.*

Thus, a stark contrast emerged between disbelief about nanobacteria and clinical evidence that coronary artery disease indicators were being reversed.

Throughout history, doctors have treated patients with compounds whose effectiveness was only later deciphered by science. In this case, it was not an untested "home remedy" that was being used. Patients were given well-known drugs that, according to Mezo, were each approved by the U.S. Food and Drug Administration and had been prescribed individually for decades, although not in this combination.

What was going on here?

A volatile yet productive mix

Competition and collaboration between Europeans and Americans has often characterized western research. European-based researchers make great discoveries, but it takes the entrepreneurial Americans to commercialize them. It is not always that way, but it has been a frequent occurrence.

The first half of this story belongs to the Europeans. Discoveries about *Nanobacterium sanguineum* began with a Finnish physician studying in America, a Turkish microbiologist who found her way to Finland, and a Hungarian researcher who later isolated the organisms in arterial plaque.

The other half of the story—a treatment for the heart disease trigger—belongs largely to this American practitioner, who, while inventing a prescription compound, crossed paths with the Europeans.

The varying cultures, temperaments, genders, scientific philosophies, and religious views of these colorful characters make a rich and volatile mix. Together they are leading the quest to conquer nanobacteria in calcification and heart disease. The characteristic that they share is unrelenting tenacity and dedication to their beliefs. The point where their lives intersect is at the fine line where research and medical practice meet.

Where old and new intersect

Mezo's treatment could not have emerged only from the halls of conventional medicine. It incorporated elements that until a few years ago had been forgotten or ignored by conformist physicians. Combining these required an understanding of conventional and "alternative" medicine, including human pathophysiology and biochemistry. Understanding this background and the context in which this therapy was developed is the first step to understanding the basis of a treatment for calcification.

Gary Mezo is not your average staid medical practitioner. He holds medical credentials and experiences that range from emergency room and family practice to indepth physiology and biochemistry. He comes from a medically streetwise background that forms the foundation for an innovative approach to medicine.

Mezo began his medical studies like every other student—in physiology and pre-med—but he says that finances intervened as they often do with medical students and he had to take a step sideways. He started by getting a Nurse Practitioner (N.P.) degree, and a Physician's Assistant (P.A.) degree.

"Back in 1975," he says, "this was a pioneering time of both professions. To survive you had to be like Avis [the car rental company that promoted itself as the underdog] and try harder."

Because many patients have been taught to believe that someone has to have the letters "M.D." after their name to be qualified to diagnose and treat disease, it is worthwhile here to give some background on the role of N.P.s and P.A.s in the medical profession.

Today, most patients in the U.S. are seen by an N.P. or P.A. at one time or another. Usually they have at least a Master's degree and additional specialized training. They diagnose, treat, prescribe medicines, deliver babies in a pinch, and do much of what M.D.s do. It is now commonly accepted for N.P.s and P.A.s to serve as primary care providers instead of an M.D.[2] It's no exaggeration to say that many medical establishments would not function effectively without N.P.s and P.A.s. They are the professional workhorses that stop overtaxed systems from falling apart. As such, N.P.s and P.A.s have practical experience that prepares them to observe the effects of diseases and drugs on patients.

"We have the desire to care, listen to patients, and be better every day," Mezo says with a characteristic air of defiant conviction, alluding to reports that label some M.D.s as being less than compassionate in their work. This comment is indicative of the close yet sometimes strained relationship between physicians and other types of licensed practitioners.

After many years of practicing, Mezo began to see an increase in the number of patients who were taking nutritional supplements—now known as "nutraceuticals"[3]—and herbal medicines.

Although they were classified as over-the-counter products, he suspected that nutraceuticals were having profound interactions with conventional medicines and effects that he couldn't assess. He did not then understand at a physiological or pharmacological level what they could do. Conventional medical training did not routinely include naturopathic studies. Therefore, most physicians were still giving their patients the standard response that such remedies were OK, based on the assumption that if they were over the counter, then they weren't a problem. He saw this trend start with vitamins, then move on to supplements for memory, and finally escalate to herbal remedies for a myriad of applications, such as lowering cholesterol. He also noted that many patients' conditions were improving with some of these alternatives.

Moreover, most of the drugs being developed by a burgeoning pharmaceuticals industry were coming from herbal sources that were then synthesized, renamed, and repackaged. So, while on one hand herbalists were often derided in conventional medicine, on the other the pharmaceuticals companies were extracting drugs from the same herbs that herbalists used, then synthesizing, renaming, and marketing them at a profit.

This contradiction spurred Mezo to study for a Ph.D. in naturopathic medicine, not so much to be an herbalist but instead to understand the chemical interactions between herbal and conventional drugs.

It was that mix of conventional and naturopathic training—then rare—that gave Mezo a new understanding of the available tools, and sent him down the road to understanding why prescription drugs were failing to treat the cause of arterial calcification in heart disease.

After many years of family and ER practice, where life and death are often hanging in the balance, his frustration grew at the number of patients who died despite surgery and a cornucopia of drugs designed to control their heart disease. None of those drugs was reversing the core problems of atherosclerosis. Few, if any of them, succeeded in getting rid of the inflammation that accompanied it.

Then one day in the late 1990s, a patient in his forties who'd had a heart attack came to Mezo's Tampa office in tears. Just a short time ago he'd led a vibrant, active life. After his heart attack though, he'd been off work for months, and his finances were in ruins. He desperately asked Dr. Mezo why no one was able to help him despite so many billions of dollars being spent on heart disease?

The world of alternative medicine had experimented with a form of therapy known as chelation that removes heavy metals from blood. (Chelation has an extensive and controversial history[4] that is summarized in Chapter 9.) Mezo perceived that chelation wasn't working as proponents said it should. The claims being made about how its pharmacological mechanisms functioned made no sense to him. Many patients appeared to get better briefly, but then they generally relapsed some time after the treatment. Also, the treatment was time consuming and expensive. On top of that, it was administered intravenously and required a visit to a doctor's office several times a week for three or four hours.

Nonetheless, at least one chemical used in chelation, EDTA (ethylenediaminetetraacetic acid), appeared to consistently show some temporary beneficial effects on patients.[5] This chemical also "sequesters," or sucks out, harmful calcium deposits; an important characteristic.

So, with his desperate forty-year-old patient in mind, Mezo began to scrutinize the conventional and alternative drug therapies for heart disease. He concluded that most were being administered in the wrong place at the wrong time of day and were missing key ingredients that might help to dissolve the calcified atherosclerotic plaque.

The first steps

Combining his background in biochemistry, physiology, medicine, and naturopathy, he devised a formula that could be administered at home by patients. It included amino acids and enzyme systems that would help to promote the opening of veins and arteries along with removal of calcium deposits from atherosclerotic plaque.

He substituted a suppository for intravenous use of EDTA. If it were used on a daily basis, he was convinced it would be safe and physiologically effective. He also filed for a U.S. patent on the process and medication formula—a step that would lead to formation of a phar-maceuticals company and foundation to develop and apply the treatment. He then had a pharmacist "compound" the preparation.

The sovereign right to compound

All pharmacists are trained as "chemists" and are often known by that title. Some of these compounding pharma-cists still do what they have done for centuries—mix in-gredients on a customized basis for individual patients. We don't hear much about this because drug companies manufacture most drugs now. Yet for prescriptions that suit the individualized needs of patients, compounding is essential because some compounds are used too seldom to be profitable for drug companies, while other com-pounds must be matched to the dosage requirements of each patient.

This compounding role of the medical chemist is usu-ally forgotten by patients who are used to seeing their pharmacist just count pills and put them in a bottle. How-ever, drug development began with chemists hundreds of years ago, and was only taken over in the 20th century by large pharmaceuticals companies.

The line between compounding and manufacturing begins at the point where the drug is put together. Ac-cording to U.S. legislation, pharmacists who compound are exempt from being regulated as manufacturers if the drug product is:

> ..."compounded for an identified individual patient based on the unsolicited receipt of a valid prescription order or a notation, approved by the prescribing prac-titioner, on the prescription order that a compounded product is necessary for the identified patient" (21 USC §353a(a)).[6]

Compounding requires a physician to write a pre-scription for their patient and deliver it to a pharmacist.

Then the pharmacist compounds the prescription for that individual patient.

Manufacturing on the other hand involves the pharmacist only in the sense that he or she takes some premanufactured pills out of a bottle and puts them into a smaller bottle for a patient. Manufacturers make pills by the millions, package them and resell them to pharmacies. Yet it's not so much the volume of pills as the serving of individualized needs that sets compounding apart from manufacturing.

Compounding had been dying out gradually over the past seventy years, but has now made somewhat of a comeback since the late 1990s due to new demands from physicians and patients for customized treatments.

Advertising and manufacturing of compounded medications are regulated in the U.S. by the Food and Drug Administration (FDA), which can force withdrawal of, or require warning labels to be put on, compounds that are specifically shown to be harmful or do not do what they are supposed to do.

If there is a documented problem with a drug that a pharmacist has compounded, then the FDA can have it taken off the market. This is the sword of Damocles that hangs over physicians and pharmacists if they compound drugs that end up being detrimental.

Gary Mezo's prescription therapy came to patients and physicians quickly because it was not a "manufactured" drug, which meant that it could be implemented without waiting years for FDA approval. Mezo adds that the ingredients in his prescription therapy—that we'll examine in Chapter 9—have each been individually approved by the FDA at one time or another, although the combination has not. "All of the components are generic and FDA approved," he explains.

Experimentation

Mezo's experience and study suggested to him that EDTA would not irritate the rectum and would be absorbed into the blood like other drugs administered by suppository. Stomach juices can destroy the effectiveness of many drugs, but rectal insertion lets them bypass the stomach and intestines, reducing the amount of drug required.

He then did something that many doctors have done but won't admit to: He tried the medication on himself. When he saw that there were no apparent ill effects, he began working with four cardiac patients who faced probable death from their illness. They had an incentive to try something new.

Much to his delight and their surprise, they started showing signs of recovery. Heart patients who were "cardiac cripples" appeared to be improving. They began walking without chest pain (angina) and reported being able to see better. In some men, their erectile function improved.

Yet these were only preliminary and sometimes anecdotal results. Mezo was worried about kidney function because EDTA is reported to cause stress on the kidneys.[7] However, the clinical measurements that he took,[8] along with kidney function began to improve in each patient. Liver function was also monitored and indicated improvement. Therefore he perceived that safety was not an immediate problem.

"Darling, I'm going to solve heart disease"

In 1998 Mezo informed his astonished wife Nancy that he was leaving his Family and Emergency Room practice to start a center to apply this new treatment. To do so he had to focus on maintaining the legally required triangle among pharmacist, physician, and patient to administer this particular treatment. Unlike mass-manufactured drugs, a drug that was "compounded" by a pharmacist had to be customized for each patient on the instruction of a physician. That was how it had usually been done before big pharmaceuticals companies arrived on the scene.

Mezo was therefore using a standard methodology to apply a revolutionary treatment. He designed a compound prescription of "old" generic medicines, using suppositories and a powder that increased the timeframe in which EDTA could work in the blood.

Yet despite this success in improving patients' conditions, his results were missing something. They suggested that the decalcification of blocked blood vessels was only proceeding to a certain point. Something was preventing it from going further. This sparked him to continue his research.

Collaboration to cut through the red tape

Being an avid reader of medical research, he had learned to exploit internet features that were allowing researchers to get newly published literature rapidly. According to him, one night around 2 a.m. the mouse led him to an obscure website in Finland, named "Nanobac Oy." It was the site of the analytical testing company that Kajander, Çiftçioglu, and some investors had started years earlier. Mezo immediately saw the missing link between his treatment and their discovery of nanobacteria. The way that they were preparing the nanobacteria was to pour EDTA on them to dissolve their calcium shells. To him, that proved why his EDTA was working on patients. The EDTA appeared to be dissolving calcified nanobacteria in hard atherosclerotic plaque, and breaking down soft plaque as he had envisaged.

Kajander and Çiftçioglu also noted on their website that tetracycline could kill nanobacteria once the shells were dissolved. Reading about this tetracycline-nanobacteria connection made Mezo see how his nanobiotic therapy could be whole. It remains that way today, he says.[9]

"Now it all made sense," he explains. "Before, cardio-vascular pathophysiology made no sense. When biochemistry rules were applied to existing cardiology concepts, they failed the litmus."

He began telephoning and finally got Neva Çiftçioglu on the phone. She was skeptical and says that she flat out didn't believe his story about treating patients with a similar method that they had been using in the lab. If true, it would catapult implementation years ahead.

After a few more discussions, Mezo was on a plane to Kuopio, Finland. The first meeting was a near-disaster. Mezo had—through an unfortunate flight delay that had worsened his jetlag—flubbed his presentation to a group of scientists and investors that Çiftçioglu had thrown him in front of half an hour after he got off the plane from a twenty-hour transatlantic trip. However, this proved to be just a temporary setback. As the three continued discussions over the next ten days they realized that they were onto something.

Kajander and Çiftçioglu were astonished to find that Mezo had circumnavigated years of what would have been regulatory red tape for them in Europe by using drugs that were individually approved by authorities and compounded as a prescription, thus avoiding the need for regulatory approval.

Yet that was only half of why Mezo had been able to apply the drug quickly. The other half was the stark reality that hundreds of thousands if not millions of persons in the U.S. alone were suffering from a terminal condition for which there was no cure—end stage atherosclerosis. They urgently needed a solution. Some of these sufferers were patients of Mezo's who had exhausted other means of treatment with other physicians and had no other hope of surviving.

Mezo saw that Kajander and Çiftçioglu, in collaboration with László Puskás from the Hungarian Academy of Sciences, had isolated the source of calcification in atherosclerotic plaque. Equally important, Kajander and Çiftçioglu had shown that once the calcium armor was removed, tetracycline could kill nanobacteria.

This requirement to simultaneously dissolve the armor and kill the nanobacteria explained why therapies that didn't specifically do both were succeeding only temporarily to improve the condition of heart patients before they started to get worse again. Nanobacteria were being exposed, and some were being excreted, but the rest were unleashed to cause havoc elsewhere in the body.

It didn't take long for the two sides to realize that collaboration could accelerate the science of heart disease and calcification treatment by years, thus saving and enhancing thousands, if not millions, of lives.

Science meets commerce

Mezo insisted that they develop a close commercial relationship, based on his justifiable concern about what happens to scientists who give their concepts away to everyone who might listen. His experience with the rough and tumble world of medical entrepreneurialism convinced him that this was critical to protect them from the fate of other pioneers who found themselves served up for lunch to predatory venture capital investors.

An added complication was that world markets had just entered into one of the worst meltdowns for technology companies in history during the stock market crash of 2000-03. Because this was going to make the job of getting capital financing difficult, it was yet another reason for their close collaboration.

Still, Çiftçioglu and Kajander weren't so easily convinced. As research scientists, they prized their academic freedom. A delicate negotiating dance began. It was a classic tension between commercial necessity and free scientific inquiry—a feature that still characterizes their cooperation.

As work on nanobacteria progresses, compromises between "open source" research and intellectual property protection for commercialization will play a defining role, as they have in the development of virtually every other drug in the marketplace today.

CHAPTER EIGHT

How Do I Know If I Have Them?

Tests have been developed to show if you're infected with nanobacteria.[1] Lab testing of randomly selected blood in Finland has shown that a significant percentage of samples turn out positive.[2] In separate analyses, every coronary heart disease patient who took the tests has also shown positive results for nanobacteria.[3]

The body develops its own defenses against nano-bacteria and produces antibodies as with other types of disease. The blood test for nanobacterial antigens and antibodies was developed by Olavi Kajander and Neva Çiftçioglu to further their research. These antigens and antibodies can be detected with the blood test known as *NanobacTEST-S* available through Nanobac Pharmaceuticals in Tampa, Florida. The test kit is sent to the patient's physician, who then draws the patient's blood and sends the sample to the closest testing lab. Nanobacterial antigens show up on a scale of one to several thousand. There is also a urine quick test *NanobacTEST-U/A,* developed by Drs. Kajander and Ilpo Kuronen in collaboration with Gary Mezo, that indicates the presence of nanobacteria by confirming nanobacterial antigen in the urine.[4]

The difficulty with depending only on the Nanobac-TESTs is that many of the dangerous nanobacteria in the body are dormant and surrounded by calcium, so they are undetectable. To quantify such calcification deposits, other methods have to be used. Mezo has developed what he calls a "nanobacterial challenge" test that he says will be evaluated in clinical studies soon.

Meanwhile, one test that gives a more graphic representation of nanobacterial infection and coronary artery disease is an Ultrafast (or Multislice) CT scan, with calcification scoring. CT Scan (or CAT scan as it's often known) is the abbreviation for Computerized Axial Tomography. It uses X-rays to scan the body from many different angles. Then it takes the information from those multiple X-rays and puts them through a computer to generate pictures of thin slices of the body. The advantage of a CT scan over a regular X-ray is that, using the same level of radiation, it can show some soft tissue and other features that X-rays miss.[5]

Calcification shows up on a CT scan because it absorbs X-rays just like bones do. That area of the film remains underdeveloped. So, if you've got calcium deposits in your heart or other organs, these will usually show up with this procedure.

In the late 1970s CT scanning was so revolutionary that its inventors were awarded the Nobel Prize. Today it is done routinely, and the accuracy is greatly improved. Without these improvements, it would be hard to see calcification in many parts of the body.

There are small risks associated with these low-dose Ultrafast CT scans. As with every method that uses X-rays, too much exposure can generate cell mutations that lead to cancer because radiation is cumulative over your lifetime. However, it is generally accepted that the benefits of an occasional CT scan usually far outweigh the risks of the X-rays. The scan is one of the best ways of "looking" at soft tissues such as the heart and lungs.[6]

Yet the problem with CT scans is that they don't show the fibrous cap and fats that gather around calcified deposits, so we still don't have the whole picture of how completely our blood vessels may be blocked.

Nonetheless, newer cardiac imaging techniques, such as Contrast MRI and Ultrasound-Enhanced CT scans, are available, and these will hopefully fill that gap. The importance of such advances is critical for heart disease patients. If physicians can see the full range of blockage in veins and arteries without using invasive techniques, then this will open the door to a world that lets them compare the effectiveness of treatments in removing and preventing such obstructions.

When taken together, the NanobacTEST and CT Heart Scan with calcium scoring are said to give convincing evidence of whether we have nanobacteria infections and how advanced the calcification is.

CHAPTER NINE

Ungumming Our Machinery

A prescription nanobiotic treatment aimed at eradicating *Nanobacterium sanguineum* in the human body has been developed by Nanobac Pharmaceuticals.[1] Its trade name is NanobacTX.

A quick refresher

Here is a reminder of the main components of heart disease to make it easier to understand how this treatment works:

First and foremost is inflammation that makes vessel walls swell. Accompanying that is plaque that coats blood vessels and is composed of a messy, complicated mix of fats (cholesterols and other lipids), calcium deposits, a fibrous cap, and globules of other complex organic materials. This combination has confounded medical doctors and pharmacists for a century or more. It is not an easy task to just clean it out.

In patients with heart disease, researchers have found nanobacteria as part of the gunk that's stuck to the insides of blood vessels. Gary Mezo theorizes that the fibrous cap is the body's attempt to wall off the nanobacterial invasion, and that this makes the problem worse by constricting arteries further.

"Up yours" to get well

The treatment is administered at home once a day in three steps: A dissolved nanobiotic powder, a suppository, and capsule.

1. The patient drinks a nanobiotic powder that has been dissolved in water or apple juice. The powder contains enzymes and amino acid systems to dissolve fibrolipid deposits and soft plaque. These components also sustain levels of disodium calcium EDTA to dissolve calcified deposits.

2. The suppository, containing a special base with the calcium-dissolving and removing (known as sequestering) agent EDTA, is inserted by the patient into the rectum before going to bed.

3. The capsule contains tetracycline hydrochloride (commonly abbreviated as tetracycline), an antibiotic that is very effective for killing nanobacteria.

According to Mezo, the three tools—nanobiotic powder, EDTA suppositories, and tetracycline—must be used together precisely as they are prescribed, to dissolve the atherosclerotic plaque and to kill the nanobacteria that are in various stages of development in the human body.

The critical nanobiotic powder component

The first job is to dissolve the fibrous cap that the immune system has constructed. The nanobiotic powder does that. It also extends the half-life of EDTA in the blood while reducing the lipid soft plaque component.

Although the precise contents of the powder remain a trade secret—just for example as the Coca Cola formula does—it basically consists of enzyme systems and amino acids.

It also tastes awful, but it can be made to taste better with apple juice.

The process is integrated rather than a linear sequence. The nanobiotic powder doesn't just strip everything off, then let the rest of the drugs work. Instead, it must be used throughout the treatment because complex deposits are mixed together in arterial plaque and throughout the circulatory system in varying thickness.

EDTA

Once that process has begun, then the EDTA, inserted by suppository into the rectum, can go to work dissolving the calcium that encases the nanobacteria.

For many years EDTA has been administered as a part of chelation therapy to remove heavy metals from the body, and in attempts to dissolve calcification of the arteries. Since there is a wealth of contradictory information in medical journals and from medical practitioners about chelation therapy, it's important to differentiate between this particular application of EDTA, and chelation as it is usually referred to.

EDTA is a colorless organic compound used to bind and extract heavy metals. It is the preferred treatment for lead poisoning and has been used for this over more than fifty years.[2] The term chelation stems from the Greek word "chele," meaning claw, as EDTA chemically grabs metal particles (such as aluminum, lead, mercury, and cadmium) and minerals (such as calcium) like a claw. Once in the blood stream, it binds to these elements. The resulting combination of EDTA, metals, and minerals is excreted from the body during urination.[3]

Some physicians who use EDTA with patients say that there are beneficial impacts to chelation in removing toxic metals, as well as other potential benefits for treating coronary artery disease.[4] Yet they add that such benefits should not be confused with questionable claims about its effects on calcification.

For example, as early as the 1950s it was hypothesized that EDTA could eliminate calcification in arterial plaque, but this is still a controversial claim.[5] Some chelation therapists maintain that their methods reduce calcification of the arteries.[6] Yet clinical studies have not shown sustainable, statistically significant decreases in atherosclerotic calcification. One trial of intravenous use of EDTA (administered by injection) claimed to show no measurable benefits for coronary artery disease patients.[7] However, that study too has been criticized for its methodology,[8] so the situation remains unclear.

Most medical associations are skeptical, and say that clinical proof about intravenous chelation's effectiveness is lacking.[9] But the National Institutes of Health (NIH) has not yet discounted its potential value. At the time of writing, a $30 million NIH study[10] was attempting to answer the question more definitively.

The NIH has summarized various theories that are suggested by EDTA chelation proponents: It might directly remove calcium from fatty plaques that block arteries, causing the plaques to disintegrate. Or it may stimulate the release of a hormone that causes calcium to be removed from plaques. Or the therapy may reduce the damaging effects of oxygen ions on the walls of the blood vessels. This might reduce inflammation and improve blood vessel function. However, the NIH concludes, "None of these theories has been well tested in scientific studies."[11]

Dr. Gary Mezo does not discount the value of chelation in removing heavy metals, but he forcefully rejects the idea that chelation can reverse calcification in coronary artery disease.

"Intravenous EDTA in combination with tetracycline will not decrease coronary calcification scores," he says. "The half-life of serum EDTA for intravenous use is twenty minutes. It will go in and be excreted through the kidneys immediately. Intravenous EDTA also happens to be given only when the subject is awake, so the metabolic rate is high and clearance is therefore rapid. If you've just eaten you've got a high load of free metabolic ions in the bloodstream from digestion."[12]

Mezo maintains that the combination of chemical processes in the body (metabolic rate), together with other changes generated by digesting food, reduces the effects of EDTA. Furthermore, he says, "EDTA suppositories combined with tetracycline at bedtime do not work any more effectively than intravenous EDTA because you don't maintain adequate EDTA serum levels.

"The powder component is critical for several reasons. First it maintains the EDTA serum levels so that they have therapeutic effect for at least twelve hours. Additionally the nanobiotic powder component has enzymes that break down that fibrotic cap and lipid layers. That allows more EDTA access to the pathological calcification buried under the fibrotic cap."

He then concludes, "Dissolving the calcification from the nanobacteria allows the tetracycline to kill them."[13]

The real differences

Mezo explains that although EDTA—as one of many components that he uses—is a sequestering agent (i.e. binds with certain materials so that they can be removed from the body), there are basic differences between his approach and what is commonly referred to as "chelation therapy":

✧ Use of EDTA chelation alone to remove arterial plaque is "incomplete and therefore risky" because it does not get rid of the underlying cause of calcification. The main risk associated with chelation is "unroofing" nanobacteria from their dormant state without using the required integrated therapies to kill them. This way they cause trouble—including risk of heart attacks—when they get loose in the blood. According to Mezo, the risks of "unroofing" nanobacteria without killing them cannot be overstated. This explains, for example, why many patients appear to get temporarily better with IV chelation, then get worse. This phenomenon is not limited to chelation. Patients who've had kidney stones pulverized or stents put into their arteries also have relapses. Many such conditions may share the same cause: Unroofed nanobacteria that then go to other parts of the body and plant themselves as "seeds" from which new dangerous growths develop. NanobacTX specifically targets nanobacteria as the underlying trigger for calcification, whereas administration of EDTA in any form alone does not.

✧ With the nanobiotic regimen, EDTA is not administered at the same time of day or in the same way as with chelation therapy. When the nanobiotic method of applying EDTA is combined with the administering of other components in the therapy, it leads to fundamental differences in the way that the human body metabolizes them.

✧ Most chelation requires that a patient go to the doctor's office several times a week for an expensive, time-consuming, and uncomfortable intravenous procedure, whereas the nanobiotic treatment is self-administered at home, eliminating medical visits that interfere with lifestyle and work.

These factors together led Mezo to reject the standard chelation treatment. Instead, he uses a combination of drugs and methods that he says lets EDTA get rid of arterial plaque, calcification, and inflammation.

Therefore, he says that if your physician hears the term "EDTA" used with the nanobiotic treatment, it is important not to jump to conclusions about this being conventionally applied chelation. He insists, "It is NOT chelation!" as commonly understood by most physicians.

Other physicians agree that Mezo's combination of EDTA with other therapies is special, but they add that whether it "is" chelation is a question of semantics.[14] They point out that chelating chemicals are a part of the therapy, but they agree that they are applied differently and do not seem to work without the treatment's many other components. Dr. James Roberts, who administers NanobacTX, also emphasizes that not one death related to chelation therapy has been reported to the Food and Drug Administration. Therefore he believes that the claim about its risks is overblown.[15]

EDTA removes heavy metals such as lead from the body. This is not essential to get at nanobacteria, but Mezo says it does help to detoxify patients, therefore enhancing the treatment's effects. As explained earlier, there is clinical evidence of such detoxifying impacts.[16]

Where the sun doesn't shine

Suppositories that are used to deliver the EDTA can be inconvenient, so why is it administered that way?

To strip the tough calcium coating from nanobacteria, a sustained blood level and reaction are required. EDTA gets torn apart by stomach acids, disrupted by metabolic activity in the daytime, and is too rapidly urinated if administered intravenously. The solution to this is to "stick it where the sun doesn't shine."

Oddly enough, Europeans have few compunctions about this, but some Americans have a phobia about putting something up their rear end. Thus, the first reaction of many patients is: Yuk! I'm not gonna do that!

However, for seriously ill patients, the choice is stark: Do or die. Furthermore, a suppository is much less discomforting and dangerous than coronary bypass surgery or being on heart drugs for the rest of their lives.

Although some patients interviewed for this book said they didn't like the idea of a suppository, they went ahead with it. So far, according to Nanobac Pharmaceuticals, most patients do not mind using the suppository, but they don't like to talk about it until after they get better.[17]

Tetracycline

Once the fibrous cap is dissipated and the calcium has been dissolved, the semi-dormant nanobacteria are exposed. Yet these "encased" nanobacteria aren't the only ones in the human body. A group of other younger nanobacteria that haven't yet encased themselves are actively emitting their toxic biofilm.

When tetracycline is administered by capsule, it immediately begins to kill the un-encased free-roaming nanobacteria, while also attacking the encased nanobacteria that have just been exposed by the EDTA. Here we see another revolution: Using an old gun to fight a new enemy. Tetracycline has been used for decades to fight a wide spectrum of infections, but it has fallen into disuse for many applications. This was due partially to resistance by bacteria, and—some argue—to the expiration of protective patents that makes the drug unprofitable for drug companies. According to Nanobac Pharmaceuticals, tetracycline is extremely effective against nanobacteria because the organism appears to be too primitive to have developed resistance to the drug. Therefore, once the cover comes off, it's helpless.

Other antibiotics are effective at killing nanobacteria, but only if the drugs are administered at levels that are toxic to humans.[18] Still others work without being toxic, but don't work as well. Tetracycline seems to have the least side effects and the highest effectiveness.[19]

The right combination and "compliance"

Once this process is underway, a battle begins in the human body. The angry "unroofed" nanobacteria come out of their dormant stage, secrete biofilm, and begin to clump together to defend themselves. This can cause trouble for cardiac patients if the special sequence of nanobiotic drugs is not applied. Too much clumping of nanobacteria may precipitate clotting and lead to a heart attack. Therefore, Mezo emphasizes that it is important to use the three weapons together precisely as they were designed; nanobiotic powder, EDTA suppositories, and tetracycline, and also to maintain your present heart drugs until your physician says that it is safe to reduce their frequency or use. And you've got to stick with it for anywhere from four months to more than a year.

Poor compliance is a major issue in medicine generally. Studies show that many patients don't take their drugs long or often enough or at the right time and that noncompliance is responsible for up to 125,000 deaths per year from cardiovascular disease.[20] Compliance isn't a small problem. It's huge.

Is occasional non-compliance harmful to the nanobiotic treatment? According to Nanobac Pharmaceuticals, accidentally missing a day or two doesn't seem to be crucial as long as the treatment is restarted and then continued as prescribed.

Bones and osteoporosis

Finally, why do nanobiotics work against calcium that afflicts our organs, yet not the calcium in our bones? Mezo says that first, the calcium that is found in our blood vessels or other parts of the body represents only a tiny fraction—less than one percent—of the total calcium in our teeth and bones. Moreover, he explains, the calcium in our teeth and bones is bound in a slightly different chemical matrix than the apatite that clogs arteries and veins.

He theorizes that his treatment may also mitigate conditions that cause loss of bone mass. Nanobacteria suck calcium out of our blood to form their protective shells. This process may interfere with the normal exchange of calcium that occurs regularly between our blood and bones. When the nanobacteria treatment eliminates the nanobacteria, they can't interfere with that process anymore. This may have implications for conditions such as osteoporosis.

Yet the real question is, does this triumvirate of pill, suppository, and powder produce measurable results in heart disease and other illnesses?

CHAPTER TEN

Does It Work?

What evidence shows if a treatment works? The first and most important is clinical: That is, measurable criteria such as blood work and calcium scores. The other is subjective, where patients report that something good is happening to them, but it hasn't been clinically verified. Some doctors also prescribe a treatment to themselves, then observe clinical and subjective results; not a generally accepted scientific practice, but sometimes done.

These excerpts from testimonials by patients are examples of what has been reported so far. As we'll see, they are far from being the only evidence of results.

February 2002.

> ...the turnaround in my health situation has been nothing short of miraculous.

> Last August, I was having some serious problems including difficulty breathing, chest pains, a rapid heart beat, lack of energy and overall, a very down feeling.

> Within six weeks after commencing the treatment, I improved dramatically and these problems resolved. I no longer have difficulty breathing, chest pains, walking distances and I am once again, positive and enthusiastic. I now feel that I have stopped aging.

...My initial spiral heart [CT] scan test done on September 6, 2001, [shows] a total calcification score of 451.7 and my second test on December 18, 2001, [shows] a total score of 348. This is a drop of 103.7 points in three and a half months, which to me is astounding.[1]

Early 2003. Heart patient with urinary problems:

Prior to treatment: Tired, sleepy, urinated about every 3-4 hours day and night, partial loss of bladder control, irritability. Swollen feet. Abnormal heart rhythm. Calcium score of 3700.

After treatment: Felt stronger more alert don't seem to need over seven hours sleep, Urinate less often and have more control over bladder. Less audible heart rhythm. Less edema. Feet and legs less swollen. Observable improvements after 6-8 months. Calcium score after eight months reduced to 1700. Has been in treatment for 13 months.

Early 2003. Heart patient with angina:

Prior to treatment: Angina. Had stents inserted after clot in heart. OK for eight or so months then angina recurred. Started to fall down for no apparent reason. Was classified as an "eleventh hour" case and recommended for open heart surgery. Did not do that but started nanobiotic treatment.

After treatment: Angina essentially gone. Ten minutes on treadmill no angina. Blood pressure generally lower. Feel better overall. Better stamina. Treatment reduced to 2 weeks on, 2 weeks off. Lost 25 pounds. Discontinued some heart drugs. Stopped nitroglycerine use. Mood has improved. Side effects looser bowels.

Early 2003. Dermatology patient with chronic rashes:

Prior to treatment. For more than 20 years had skin rashes. Dermatologists prescribed creams. They would work for a short time then another rash came. Had rash all over body that "itched and itched."

After treatment. After first month of treatment noticed improvement. After three months, was free of rash. Then cut down treatment to three times a week, then two. Then stopped all treatment. Then the rashes started again. Took treatment for 16 days and it cleared up. Now takes three treatments at the beginning of each month. Gums are in better shape.

At first had some diarrhea and flatulence but that went away.[2]

Mid-2003. Heart patient who is an MD allergist:

Before treatment: Intense jaw and neck pain while exercising. Obstruction of right coronary artery. Couldn't walk up two flights of stairs "without getting in trouble". Stent was put in but then blocked.

After treatment: Calcium score dropped by at least 25 percent. Pain gone during exercise. Dropped back treatment to two weeks per month, then stopped, but continues with his regularly prescribed heart drugs. No negative side effects. A cataract in his eye has disappeared.

"If this is as good as it looks on paper right now and [knowing that] I'm feeling as good as I have felt in the past year and a half, for example my stent should have plugged over and it hasn't...I just have to think that there has to be something going on that's a positive situation at least for me."[3]

Together these testimonials make a compelling case. Yet, when we consider such results, we also have to understand that calcification is the toughest thing to get rid of compared to inflammation, clotting, and soft plaque in atherosclerosis. Hard calcium deposits are the last thing to go. According to the researchers and physicians who work with the treatment, this is why patients first begin to show improvements in their blood and in signs of inflammation. Then only later do physical indicators of calcification reduction begin to show.

Thus, although calcification appears to be at the core of the problem, it is also among the last of the measurable heart disease indicators to be reversed. This may help to explain why some of the first improvements are seen in patients' general energy levels long before their calcium scores start to drop.

The marathoner cardiologist

Dr. James C. Roberts practices what he preaches by maintaining a rigorous exercise regimen. He runs about forty miles a week. Such determination perhaps explains why he is also one of the few mainstream cardiologists who has successfully treated heart patients with what was once seen as an alternative therapy known as Enhanced External Counter Pulsation (EECP). In plain terms, that's bypassing blocked arteries with pressure blasts that open up small arteries to improve blood flow.

EECP is a good example of a therapy that relieves heart disease symptoms for very ill heart patients and improves their chances for avoiding a heart attack, but does not cure the disease. With this therapy, pneumatic cuffs are placed over the patient's lower extremity, then inflated and deflated repeatedly. This drives oxygenated blood backwards from the lower parts of the body into the heart. That in turn increases pressure between the open arteries and those that are blocked by heart disease. The pressure stimulates formation of small natural "bypasses." That is, the body expands its own tiny arteries. The therapy is often used for patients who are considered to be "too far gone" to undergo stent implants or bypass surgery.

According to Roberts, EECP is a low risk, non-invasive procedure that can be done quickly outside the hospital. A full course of therapy typically involves 35 one-hour treatments done over seven weeks. The cost of EECP is a fraction of bypass surgery or angioplasty (widening the artery with a balloon-like device). EECP is covered by most commercial insurers, as well as the major Health Maintenance Organizations (HMO) that serve Roberts' local area, and by Medicare.[4]

Roberts is the Medical Director of the EECP Center of Toledo, Ohio. He has seventeen years of experience in cardiology. He doesn't like losing patients, especially to premature death. Yet in his part of the practice where the worst cardiac cases end up, it's a brutal fact of life. That's why he started looking at therapies outside of the conventional ones that had been only of limited use to his patients.

Since 1997 he successfully treated hundreds of patients with EECP. Yet he still faced a problem.

If patients have advanced blockage in their lower extremities, or don't have one good artery left from which to grow natural bypasses, or they suffer from irregular heartbeat (arrhythmia) or heart failure, then it is far more difficult to successfully apply EECP.

"Unfortunately, half of the patients referred to us by other cardiologists have one of these four complicating features. Now we can stabilize the cardiac rhythm with drugs, and heart failure can be compensated for medically, but if all three arteries of the heart are blocked, or if there is poor blood flow to the legs—well, then we're stuck. We can try as hard as we can and the patient can try as hard as he/she can, but these patients don't get a good result. This is upsetting, as to these patients, EECP was their 'last hope.'"[5]

In other words, many of his patients were suffering and dying; a sad but not unusual phenomenon in end stage heart disease victims.

Then in May 2001 Roberts came across the work of Dr. Mezo, who theorized, based on a ninety patient pilot study, that the stuff plugging arteries results from long-standing infection by an organism that can be treated.

Roberts says that initially, "I got a good laugh at Dr. Mezo's expense—what a ridiculous theory. I 'knew' that atherosclerosis was due to high cholesterol and the other risk factors that we (allegedly) knew about."

But Mezo supported the claim. In his pilot study he explained that ninety patients were treated and their 'calcium scores' fell.[6] These scores, taken from rapid X-rays of the arteries, measure dangerous buildups that cause heart attacks (see Glossary for more details).

Roberts was experiencing what many physicians across America were going through—a disbelieving but fascinated reaction to what appeared to be a crazy claim: Coronary calcification was being reversed.

Like other doctors, he also had to overcome a deep discomfort with prescribing a drug whose contents he was not 100 percent aware of. Components of the nanobiotic powder were being kept a trade secret. He also wasn't happy with what he saw as some overly optimistic claims by the treatment's developers.

Yet the alternatives—continued pain and certain death among his patients—drove him to tell them about the treatment and suggest that they try it.

As he treated his patients, Roberts was among the first to discover that the clinical signs in patients started to improve. They didn't just improve slightly; they improved remarkably. For example, some patients who had no pulse in their feet due to arterial blockage started to have one again.

Roberts made a convincing argument for the treatment by publishing the case histories of some patients on his website.[7] The results include CT Heart Scan images that show indicators of calcium reduction, plus other test results that clinically demonstrate improved cardiovascular function.

Some of the material contained in the next pages is more technical than in the rest of this book because it describes clinical evidence that has been observed by Roberts as a practicing physician. We included a few of his observations so that patients and their physicians might get a more complete view of what he has seen.

Roberts made an important discovery: In some cases, calcium scores didn't change in the first course of treatment, but patients still exhibited clinical signs of improvement.

Here are excerpts from those case histories. Some of the language is technical. For unfamiliar terms, please refer to the Glossary in the back.

(Note: These passages are paraphrased, and in some parts quoted from Dr. Roberts' website[8] and correspondence. Roberts' case studies are excellent introductions to various applications of the treatment. See the "nanobacterium sanguineum" portion of his website at www.heartfixer.com)

Patient MP: Atherosclerosis everywhere

MP had severe vascular disease. In 1992 she underwent bypass surgery on several arteries, followed by multi-drug treatment. That went on until 2001 when she began to experience chest pains once or twice daily. She suffered from severe blockage of the arteries in her lower extremities and had no pulse in her feet. She also had a kidney cyst and narrowing in the arteries to the kidneys, brain, and left arm. She had atherosclerosis everywhere and wasn't a candidate for further medical procedures. With her severe disease, she also wasn't a candidate for EECP (a treatment described earlier).

Roberts says that had he seen MP two months before, he would have turned her away as untreatable. Once having heard of NanobacTX, he put her on it.

Two months into treatment MP's chest pains improved, a detectable pulse on the top of the foot developed, and Roberts began EECP. After four months MP's chest pain went away. The left foot pulse was now full, and MP's blood flow to the lower extremities improved. Roberts was also able to discontinue a drug treatment to help the kidneys work because her kidney function had also improved.[9]

Patient BD: He was treated with NanobacTX, and his CT scores did not drop in blocked blood vessels, but he improved nonetheless

BD doesn't smoke, his lipids and blood sugar are under control, and he exercises, but his Lipoprotein "A" ("really bad" cholesterol) is in the top five percent of the population. This type of cholesterol is designed by nature to be a repair particle. Unfortunately it also tries to "repair" vessels that have had surgery, blocking them.

In 1991 BD had a heart attack. Angiography demonstrated narrowing of the arteries, so grafts were placed in them. BD returned six months later with a second heart attack, due to closure of one graft. In 1994 another graft closed down, so angioplasty was performed. Chest pain recurred in late 1999 because the angioplastied artery had renarrowed. BD was left with only one open artery. EECP was carried out and worked well, but chest pain returned in 2001.

BD lived out of town, so travel was an issue. EECP and other therapies require daily visits to a doctor's office. Since anti-nanobacterial therapy does not, it could be done at home.

BD tolerated the nanobiotic well, but his CT score rose after four months. He was disappointed, but he agreed to two more months of treatment. His score then fell, but was still above where it had been at the start.

At first look this might suggest that the nanobiotic didn't work. Yet BD's chest pain had fully resolved for the first time in years. His "good" cholesterol (HDL) rose ten points, and his "really bad" cholesterol dropped by eleven. His ability to exercise increased measurably, as did other clinical factors. So from a perspective that excluded calcium scores, nanobiotics were working.

Why such a mismatch between the CT findings and the patient's clinical, laboratory, and stress test findings? It is worth exploring, because Roberts often sees this when treating patients with long-standing atherosclerosis and bypass grafts. Here are some of the reasons that he suggests:

> ...In these long-standing coronary disease patients with dense calcification, it may be difficult for the radiologist to determine where calcification ends in (one part of the heart) and where it begins in (another). The radiologist who reads your first scan may not be the radiologist who reads your second, and the cut-off point is a little subjective, and this can lead to "shifts" in the calcium scores from one vessel to another.

> Sometimes, but not always, a metal clip is used to affix the bypass graft to the bypassed artery; this will show up on the Ultrafast CT scan as calcium, the same situation as with the coronary stent—this confuses the reading. [10]

Then there is what Roberts describes as the *Blind Alley* effect in patients who've had grafts.

> The artery is open only over its initial one third, and thus it receives little flow. The artery is occluded in more than one location; portions may be "isolated."

> If our goal is only to decalcify the coronary artery and make the CT scan look better, then we have a problem, as we aren't going to be able to get much NanobacTX into these blind alley regions which typically contain the heaviest calcification. We may not, *at least not within four months*, significantly alter the natural history of calcification progression in (these) regions.

We get plenty of treatment into (other) vessels and into the microcirculation, but these regions don't contain much calcium, so calcium score wise, we have little to show for our work and the patient's efforts.

We are certainly getting NanobacTX into the bypass grafts, but the CT scanners available today aren't able to calcium score the bypass grafts, so any improvement in graft wall calcium goes "unrecognized."

Thus when we treat post-bypass patients with NanobacTX their symptoms decrease, their lab values improve, and their stress parameters increase, but the calcium scores over their bypassed vessels may not change—they may even go up, even though the patient is getting better.

For these reasons, I am now typically not obtaining CT scans on my post-bypass patients. They have coronary atherosclerosis, so I know that they have a vascular wall Nanobacterial infection, and a follow-up scan is often misleading, so why not save the patient some money, and treat them based on symptoms, stress test, and laboratory parameters, which do seem to reflect what it actually going on in the patient?[11]

In a later case history of another patient Dr. Roberts adds this important finding about the usefulness of tests for diagnosing progress:

We know that CRP (C-Reactive Protein), the best marker of vascular wall inflammation, is also our best predictor of who will and who will not develop coronary disease, and who will have an adverse coronary event, or experience a complication or recurrence of disease following angioplasty, stent placement, or bypass surgery. Statin cholesterol lowering drugs, antioxidants, and fish oil all have been shown to lower CRP a little, but not like this. We typically see a pronounced drop in CRP when we treat cardiovascular patients with NanobacTX, and it may just be that vascular wall inflammation, due to *Nanobacterium sanguineum*, is the culprit underlying this ominous inflammatory marker.[12]

Patient MJ: The Case of the "Up-Down Phenomenon"

Among the results identified by Roberts and others is an apparent *increase* in calcium and antibody test scores in the early stages of nanobacteria treatment, followed by a decrease later. It has to be emphasized here that there is some difference of opinion among physicians who prescribe nanobiotics as to whether and how much calcium scores actually go up when patients are being initially treated. Some argue that the rise in the score can be attributed to inaccuracies in older technologies that were first used to score patients. Roberts acknowledges this but still maintains that he and other physicians have noticed increases in calcium scores in some patients. He says that one explanation for the increase is that nanobacteria may be able to somehow hide themselves temporarily from the treatment, and in that interval re-calcify. But he emphasizes this is a guess. The outcome of the scoring discussion will be significant for understanding how calcium scoring and the process of decalcification work. Regardless of that, there is agreement that at least antibody scores do seem to show a temporary increase. Furthermore, the physicians also agree that short-term calcium scoring may be less important to patients' well-being than reductions in other measurable heart disease symptoms that are reliably determined with bloodwork.

> MJ's four month score increase (after a four month course of NanobacTX) from 1347 to 3070 is way beyond the natural history of coronary artery calcification (20-80% progression per year, depending on the study), so it must be a treatment related effect. The score got worse, but MJ got better—how can we explain this? [13]

With ongoing therapy, MJ's score fell steadily, until after fourteen months it was at 1209, and according to Roberts, clinically he was "doing great."[14]

(Note: Roberts qualifies the below observations by stating that they are based on his experience treating patients, his understanding of the scientific literature, and conversations with Drs. Mezo and Çiftçioglu. He emphasizes that he can't back up everything that he says here with a scientific study.)

> MJ's case…serves as the most extreme example to date of the Up-Down Effect….How, at least in theory, could we make the patients worse with NanobacTX? How could we aggravate their vascular wall Nanobacterial infection?

> …When we dissolve (nanobacteria's) calcific shelters with EDTA and "unroof" them, the Nanobacteria feel threatened. They respond by…(increasing) their growth rate and elaborating copious amounts of biofilm. The large volume of biofilm goo which now surrounds the few Nanobacterial cell bodies begins to lightly calcify….

> If we took a CT scan at this point, we would score calcium over a large area, even though there are relatively few live Nanobacteria present. If we waited for the biofilm to condense into shelters, then the area involved with calcification would condense.

> If we kill the now non-sheltered and thus vulnerable Nanobacteria with tetracycline, then new shelters will not form up. The Nanobacteria will be eradicated and the calcium score will drop….

> …Coronary calcification is rarely evenly distributed within your arteries; this means that different arteries were infected at different times and will have different calcium scores when NanobacTX therapy is initiated. Thus each artery will demonstrate the Up-Down Phenomena at different time points. Thus, at 4 months, we may see…a gross Up-Down Phenomena, as in patient MJ.

> We are winning the battle and the patient is getting better, and with further therapy the patients will further improve and their calcium score will eventually fall, but at half-time, judging by the CT score alone, it looks as if the Nanobacteria have the upper hand—

but they don't; this is simply the Up-Down Phenomenon.[15]

The observations of physicians like Roberts were invaluable in establishing the benefits and side effects of
the nanobiotic treatment. These doctors took a leap with
their patients who were "too far gone" for other treatment. In so doing they laid their reputations on the line.

That same motivation to treat "untreatable" patients
sparked other more conservative cardiologists to look at
Mezo's therapy.

The cardiologist's cardiologist

On the wall of Dr. Benedict Maniscalco's waiting room is
a framed certificate identifying him as being voted one of
the "Best Doctors In America." He *is* the medical estab-
lishment; a conservative cardiologists' cardiologist who
doesn't take chances with his patients without sober consideration.

Maniscalco is well known in Tampa, Florida, where he
has treated tens of thousands of cardiac patients. He was
instrumental in developing cardiology facilities in the Tampa
Bay area. In his own words he likes to stick to proven
remedies, but also keeps "an open mind" to new approaches.[16] He's no alternative medicine maverick.

Yet he also knows that cardiology is ultimately a losing battle in that the patient always ends up dying of
heart disease or complications arising from it. Normally
every cardiologist considers his or her work successful if
the relentless progress of heart disease is slowed, or in
special cases arrested. Various drugs and diet regimens
reduce the likelihood of heart attack, and some treatments seem to prevent the formation of clots. Yet as
we've seen, the progress of calcification and atherosclerosis (or hardening of the arteries, as most of us know it)
has never been properly explained, understood by medical experts, or reversed before.

As a self-confessed skeptic of new heart treatments, he explains what inspired him to try the nanobiotic treatment with his patients:

"We've known for 200 years that atherosclerotic plaque was an inflammatory process. And we've always thought and been taught that calcium in a plaque was simply the point in the inflammatory reaction in which the calcium deposition occurred. Maybe it was there to strengthen the repair process.

"In the past 10-15 years there have been many investigations into the lining of the arteries and plaque, and we have investigated a number of infectious agents. Those investigations by a number of major institutions around the world clearly tell us that infectious agents play a significant role and may cause the initial injury that starts the inflammation that leads to the plaque.

"We have had large scale clinical trials in this country in which we've used antibiotics to treat certain organisms that we thought to be the leading pathogen: Mainly *Chlamydia pneumoniae*, and the clinical outcomes have not been encouraging because we've not seen a significant difference.

"Gary Mezo presented to me his knowledge of *Nanobacterium sanguineum*. Çiftçioglu and Kajander demonstrated that *Chlamydia* has a cross-reactive antigen with nanobacteria, which was immediately a very enticing thought that, gee, we're detecting what we think is *Chlamydia* but it may be something else.

"Then I read the paper that Dr. Puskás of Hungary had tried to get published unsuccessfully, in which he isolated nanobacteria from atherosclerotic plaque.

"So think of my reaction in this way: I've been a cardiologist for almost 30 years and I haven't cured anyone. I have been involved with bringing relief to thousands of patients and providing state of the art cardiology diagnosis and treatment services, but "cure" is another thing. So when you look at the thought that there is possibly a way to approach a plaque, break it down, re-move the offending pathogen, and eliminate that plaque, then that's an astounding thought."[17] (Note: For a further explanation in Maniscalco's words, see the Foreword.)

Until then, the idea that a coronary heart disease trigger might be found, then reversed was not in the realm of experience. For cardiologists such as Maniscalco, it meant possible salvation from a distressing occupational hazard: Watching patients whom they'd known for years die of an incurable disease.

A clinical trial

In the medical and scientific world, clinical trials are essential, while anecdotal results are just that: Anecdotal. No regulatory agency accepts anecdotal evidence as proof. They also won't pay much attention to clinical evidence, such as that presented by Dr. James Roberts, unless these data are part of a rigorously controlled, independently monitored study. Patients can be raised from the dead and dance a jig on their graves, but this alone is insufficient proof when it occurs outside the confines of an orthodox, controlled study.

There are good reasons for this skepticism. Treatments that seem to help patients get better may be influenced by something that the physician has not considered. On top of that, despite the regulation of medicine by many authorities, mistakes are often made and bad practices still abound.[18] The best way to minimize these and achieve accurate results is to conduct studies under strictly supervised conditions, with independent oversight. Therefore, to guarantee risk/benefit analysis and protect patient rights, guidelines for conducting and interpreting clinical trial studies are agreed with independent agencies such as Institutional Review Boards (IRBs).

Controversy continues in the medical world over how much study is required prior to a new treatment being brought to the marketplace, especially in the cases of patients who have no other alternative except death.

Regulatory agencies delay bringing trial drugs to market until they have undergone time-consuming, exhaustive studies. Meanwhile, thousands die. Pressure to bring drugs to market earlier increases as wealthy and famous individuals start keeling over. An example of this occurred with AIDS.

The depth of this controversy is profound, especially in America where patients now make more visits annually to complementary and alternative medicine (CAM) healers than to medical doctors.[19] In 1998 the National Center for Complementary and Alternative Medicine (NCCAM) was started, signifying the new legitimacy of alternative treatments. Alongside this, declining profits from conventional treatment, and insurers' increasing readiness to cover CAM, have led more than one hundred reputable medical centers to start alternative medicine clinics. Some offer therapies that have been verified through few, if any, clinical trials. Yet they are administered nonetheless due to what some say have been convincing anecdotal results.[20]

Such pressure has brought a more lenient attitude towards the types of studies being done on treatments for patients who have no other choices. For example, the highest form of test results verification is seen as the control group or "double blind" approach, where one group is given a placebo with no drug while the other is given the real thing, and the researchers testing the results also do not know which group they are dealing with. The drawback of such an approach is that it is expensive and lengthy, leading to delays in bringing products to terminally ill and pain-ridden patients.

Therefore, studies that do not use such "blind" verification are in some cases allowed as a first step to broader introduction of a treatment. Still, there is one caveat; it must be shown that the treatment does not harm, or that it at least does less harm than the disease that it is aimed at controlling.

At the same time a contrary trend has emerged that makes the task of carrying out studies more arduous. With the "publish or die" syndrome running rampant in the academic community, pressure to produce early results is enormous, and many mistakes have been made. Scandals have erupted over the accuracy and safety of studies. A few years ago major research institutions such as Johns Hopkins lost their federal funding when patients participating in studies fell ill or died unexpectedly.[21]

As evidence of short cutting and questionable results mounted, regulatory and research agencies started being more stringent about what is a "study" and how it is conducted.

Nanobac Pharmaceuticals knew that clinical trial evidence from reputable sources was required to convince skeptics about the legitimacy of the nanobiotic prescription and to repel attacks by critics. Dr. Mezo saw that such work had to be carried out in concert with a recognized Institutional Review Board (IRB) oversight agency.

An earlier NanobacTX "Atherosclerotic Calcification Eradication Study" and a NanobacTX Pilot had been done, but these weren't under the monitoring of an outside authority. This led Mezo to approach a high level group of physicians and clinical trial experts to measure and validate results in a formal IRB clinical study. Thus began a clinical trial supervised by Dr. Maniscalco under rules established by the Western Institutional Review Board (WIRB).[22]

"This was the first study of a nanobacteria treatment to be done under the auspices of an Institutional Review Board," Maniscalco explains. "We wrote a protocol specifically to be followed that was submitted to the Western IRB. The purpose of involving such a review agency is first to protect the patient to make sure that safety precautions are taken and that, for example, patients don't

accidentally die due to an inadequately supervised protocol. Secondly, the agency insures that studies are done
according to pre-established guidelines and ethical con-
siderations."[23]

How it started

Because the patient base of the clinical study was relatively small, it's important to understand what such an
analysis may or may not prove under the parameters
established.

Dr. Maniscalco says that when he and Dr. Mezo first
met, he was intrigued by the aim of Mezo's pilot study
that had already been done on a few patients who had
calcification: "…If those calcifications mean 'arterial plaque',
then if it's true that increasing amounts of calcium mean
increasing amounts of plaque, then if it can be reversed,
that would be a phenomenal discovery."[24]

Mezo had told Maniscalco that this was exactly what
had happened in his earlier pilot study. After Maniscalco
investigated the literature on nanobacteria, he agreed to
do the clinical trial under the auspices of an IRB.

The main purpose of the trial was to analyze and
validate the "before and after" clinical symptoms of patients with heart disease who were treated with the
nanobiotic. A main detection method was High Speed CT
Heart Scan that shows the level of calcium in coronary
arteries. Maniscalco talked to some of his patients who
had coronary disease with a lot of calcification in their
arteries and enlisted them for the trial.

Tests for nanobacteria antibodies and antigens were
taken, along with tests such as electrocardiograms, CRP,
cholesterol, and other indicators that focus on inflammation in heart disease. Then Maniscalco put them on the
nanobiotic and started monitoring changes.

"The intended end point was to determine whether a
four month treatment with NanobacTX would lead to a

drop in the calcium score as recorded in technology called Electron Beam Computed Tomography (EBCT) or Helical Ultrasound Tomography (HCT)." (Note: Both methods are used for heart scanning.) "We screened about 130 patients. We wanted to have a hundred complete. We ended up with 77 patients who completed it."

An outside review committee of cardiologists then was chosen. "It was their job to confirm that data was collected, that it is in fact what I said it is, and that the protocol is followed properly."[25]

Results so far

Statistical results are not being made available until they are published in a recognized journal, but Dr. Maniscalco has made general observations that can be relayed here, as discussed in the Foreword to this book: "I've observed patients that have had clear changes in their calcium scores. That in itself is remarkable."[26]

"In four months we've noted patients who have marked variations in their (nanobacterial) antigen and antibody scores. We had patients coming into the study with an antigen of zero and we started treating them. As we break down the calcium, suddenly the antigen level goes shooting up. Then we treat them and a few months later it's down again. That can only mean to me that we're liberating the source of the antigen from a plaque, and subsequently it becomes detectable and we're killing it. And the antigen falls to zero.

"Along with that we've noticed that some patients who have limited functional capacity can double or quadruple [theirs]. For instance, one lady on the treadmill could walk maybe six to nine minutes and now she walks 45 minutes to an hour.

"We've noticed patients whose symptoms limited their exercise, but now whose symptoms went away. I have a patient who came in with severe angina of the legs, no pulses in his lower extremities, and we treated him and the angina went away and the pulses came back.

"The other thing that's astounding to me, that I've never seen in thirty years, is that pulses are zero then they come back."

This was the same phenomenon noted earlier by Dr. James Roberts.

"There was no ill effect on kidney," Maniscalco adds. "No ill effect on liver. No ill effect on bone marrow that I could tell by looking at blood work. And there seemed to be pretty much a strong effect on lowering cholesterol, raising HDL ("good" cholesterol) and lowering LDL ("bad" cholesterol) beyond the [effects of] the therapy that patients were already on.

"In general I've learned that patients feel more energetic and better after they've been on it for a while. We've seen decreases in calcium scores, which can only mean that we're decreasing plaque. We've seen fluctuations in antigen (and) antibodies which mean that we're liberating the bacteria and killing them. We've seen changes in functional capacity in symptoms that can't be explained in any other way than in the fact that we treated them."

After the study was completed, Maniscalco continued the treatment, especially with some of his patients who hadn't shown as convincing results: "I'm noticing now that even those whose scores didn't change much in four months continue to get better and their scores are falling precipitously after the trial was over."

Duration and side effects

Side effects are discussed further in the next chapter, but Dr. Maniscalco says that in the study he observed this: "The only major side effect that made us have to withdraw (one) patient was (an) allergic reaction to a component of the treatment."

He has reached his own conclusions about how long the treatment needs to be applied to be effective for seriously ill patients: "This is not a treatment that takes one month or four months. This is a long-term treatment. Something that hopefully won't be a year or two all the time, but for people with advanced disease it's going to take quite a long time. Because the more plaque you have the longer you've had the disease. We know that it progresses at forty percent a year so it's not going to all go away in four months or eight months."[27]

Furthermore, as Dr. James Roberts had also reported, for a few patients it seems that "nothing happened." Why do some show no improvements? Does it just take the treatment more time to work for them?

Still other patients had to drop out of the study due to an over-sensitivity to tetracycline. Will there be another solution for them?

Then there is the suppository. "The toughest part of this whole thing is that the compound includes a suppository," says Dr. Maniscalco, "and we're not used to using a suppository except with our children. The suppository has some local side effects that are disturbing to patients, but after a two week period usually things pretty much settle down."

Does Maniscalco think that we might eventually get around the suppository? "When big pharma [the big pharmaceutical companies] has a will, they have a way and there will be a solution to the suppository."[28]

A patient who participated in the trial

The authors interviewed a small number of patients who participated in the first clinical trial of NanobacTX shortly after the trial was completed. Here is one patient's story:

In 1989 JK had a three-way bypass and ten years later a quadruple bypass. In his whole life he'd never had high cholesterol or high blood pressure. Just like about a third of heart patients, he had very few of the traditional telling indicators. Yet heart disease killed both his parents and his grandparents.

"Like most people that go through heart treatment I got a lot of books and read everything I could about [conventionally accepted causes and treatments]. Frankly none of it made a lot of sense. The typical science for coronary arteries didn't seem to fit me, and I also found many places where people who did fit [the profile] didn't have the disease. It just wasn't consistent in my layman's mind.

"I've always been pretty active. I used to be very active in racing cars, and I raced motorcycles when I was a young man. I was an avid golfer.

"I got to the point where I couldn't do a lot of those things anymore. I certainly couldn't race cars. I ended up with angina pain after two or three laps in the car. Playing golf I could not walk the course anymore without angina pain, and that's what really finally convinced me to have the second bypass surgery.

"About three months after the surgery I was on a treadmill and one of my arteries collapsed while I was on the treadmill. I just didn't have the energy and the whole lifestyle wasn't as good as it had been.

"Dr. Maniscalco came to me and said, 'There's this experimental treatment that you might fit.'"

So JK started the treatment. After Maniscalco gave him literature, he found some more and read about it himself.

"Right off the bat there was no noticeable difference except that the indigestion was a problem. That went away after about three weeks. After a couple of months I just...felt better. I got back to the point where I could walk 18 holes, no problem. I even played 36 holes one day with no problem. I'm racing the car now. I just got back from three weeks on a motorcycle [tour] in the Alps. Not a single problem.

"Before the treatment I was taking Toprol and aspirin, and Diltiazem (to control blood pressure and chest pain). When I started the treatment Dr. Maniscalco added Foltx (a folic acid and B Vitamin supplement), and Niacin.

"I was on the treatment for six months and we did a Heart Scan at the beginning and at the end of that. Two years after bypass surgery (before he started the treatment) I had one artery that was 30 percent blocked, and [now] at the end of the treatment I have zero blockage."

It appeared as though the treatment actually reversed the disease process. It also had some interesting side effects:

"One of the things that really felt better was arthritis pain. I don't have a severe case...I have it in my back and my neck, but my back didn't hurt anymore. My neck didn't hurt.

"I've had kidney stones in the past. Starting about the fifth month, I passed a kidney stone, and about a week later I passed another kidney stone. I went to the urologist and had an X-ray done and had four more kidney stones. I told my urologist about the treatment and he pooh-poohed it as hocus pocus, but I gave him the website and he came back later and said it looked interesting."

JK decided to continue with the treatment on a part time basis and does it 3-4 times a week. "I'm not religious about it now."

"I am a convert. I believe in the treatment and I'm going to do what my doctor recommends."[29]

He hasn't discussed getting off his other medicines yet, but he wants to.

Once again, it is important to note that JK is one of the patients who participated in the independently monitored clinical study, so his impressive results can be confirmed with a high level of confidence.

The case of Dr. C.

Just after Dr. Maniscalco had made a presentation at a conference of allergists to explain preliminary results of the NanobacTX ACES II Cardiology Study trial, he was approached by retired physician Dr. C.

Various physicians have prescribed the nanobiotic for themselves, but the case of Dr. C. was especially poignant because although the Nanobac Pharmaceuticals staff had dealt with his prescription as they do with thousands of patients, Drs. Maniscalco and Mezo did not know about it personally. As such this came as an unsolicited response from a physician with whom they were not familiar.

Dr. C. says that his condition is the classic example of the adage, "You can pick your friends but not your relatives," because he had a history of heart disease in his family.

His case was in some ways typical. Knowing the history of the affliction in his family, he had been careful about his diet and exercise, hoping to dodge the coronary bullet. Nonetheless, one day while he was golfing, he began to feel a pain in his neck. He tried to ignore it, but some weeks later it came back. When he consulted with a cardiologist friend of his, he was immediately scheduled for an emergency angioplasty where a blocked artery was "ballooned" and a stent inserted to let the blood begin flowing. Some time later the neck pain returned and, as is often the case, it was discovered that the stent had blocked, so the artery had to be reopened.

At an earlier meeting of allergists, Dr. C. had heard about the nanobiotic treatment, so he decided to prescribe it for himself. After six months, his calcium score dropped by at least a quarter. He says that it may have been more than that because, as explained earlier, there are still technical problems ascertaining the level of calcification in a stent when a CT scan has difficulty differentiating between the stent and calcium. Nonetheless, the one-quarter reduction was statistically significant. His stent had not reblocked at that point.

Besides the calcium score reduction, a cataract in one of Dr. C.'s eyes disappeared, leading to cancellation of planned surgery to remove it. When his ophthalmologist searched for the cataract and couldn't find it, he apparently remarked that he'd never seen such a phenomenon. It was a remarkable occurrence.

In an interview with the authors, Dr. C. said that he experienced no side effects from the treatment except having to be "close to a bathroom" in the morning.[30] He added that he would recommend the treatment.

CHAPTER ELEVEN

Caution:
It May Not Be For Everybody

The treatment for calcification is undoubtedly encouraging. Yet, according to Dr. James Roberts, who has some of the most extensive experience with nanobiotics, there is a qualification:

> Despite all the promising early news about this nanobiotic, it should not be considered a panacea. First, it needs to be tested in larger clinical trials of longer duration before I'm confident of its usefulness. Second, "fluffing" the calcified plaque to allow the tetracycline ample penetration could possibly precipitate angina. Such was the case for one of my patients, who had to withdraw from the study.

> For now, I would treat those patients with very high calcium scores or those with angina who have a poor quality of life and are running out of options. This is where the real beauty of nanobiotics for anti-nanobacterial treatment lies—providing one more card for us physicians to play when the stakes are the highest. Otherwise, there's little we can do when someone's vessels are clogged beyond repair.

> Perhaps we'll eventually discover new combinations of procedures.[1]

The good and the bad

According to Nanobac Pharmaceuticals and some of the independent physicians who have prescribed the treatment, there have been good and bad clinical and anecdotal results observed in patients. These do not occur in every patient, but rather are varying results that have been observed among some patients. That's to say, not everyone is going to experience each of the results shown in Figure 9.

Risks

As emphasized throughout this book, every patient should consult with a qualified physician prior to doing any treatment, and that also applies to this one.

The real and perceived risks of using a treatment for nanobacteria vary depending on your condition. For those who are among the tens of millions suffering from life-threatening circulatory disease, "relative risk" takes on a different meaning compared to the risk for a healthy person who is at only the beginning stages of heart disease and is not slowed or crippled by it. Patients who have shown the most dramatic improvements are those who are worst off. There is a historical reason for this: The treatment was first tried on those who had exhausted other available means. Dr. Mezo had made the decision to treat the inoperable, the "cardiac cripples," that is, those heart disease victims who had no other options. He surmised that if they improved, then so would those with less severe disease. For these severely ill individuals the relative risks of nanobacteria treatment compared to the risks of dying from heart disease are minuscule.

Yet for someone who is not showing symptoms of a calcification-related disease, then there may be cause for thought, because the treatment hasn't been around long enough to show its warts.

The Good:	**Clinical observations:** Improvements have been recorded in: Ability to exercise Blood pressure Calcium scores Diabetes symptoms "Good" and "bad" cholesterol Inflammation indicators such as C-reactive protein, erythrocyte sedimentation rate, fibrinogen, and white blood cell count Pulse Triglicerides Stress tests
	Anecdotal observations: Improvements have been noted in: Age (liver) spot reduction Angina symptoms Arthritic conditions (bursitis and tendonitis) Chronic prostatitis or E.D. Cognitive abilities and/or memory Eyesight General sense of well being Kidney stones being passed Psoriasis, eczema, lichen planus or scleroderma Sex drive
The Bad:	**Clinical observations:** Abdominal cramping, loose stools and occasionally wet gas with symptoms usually subsiding with continued treatment after 7-10 days Tetracycline caused mild stomach upset and gas Rectal irritation from the suppositories in patients with hemorrhoids
	Anecdotal observations: Difficulty complying with the regimen Rare cases of angina in patients with a history of angina, that usually goes away after 1-2 months of treatment

Figure 9: Clinical and anecdotal observations from administering the NanobacTX treatment

Let's have a brief look at each of these risks and who says what about them:

Tetracycline. At one time this was on the front line of the miracle drug revolution due to its ability to kill a wide spectrum of bacteria. Then resistance set in and its effectiveness diminished, so it is not as widely prescribed now. Most individuals have no trouble with the drug aside from mild stomach upset that usually diminishes after a few days. A rare percentage of the population are allergic, and for them it's a rough ride. Some patients get severe headaches. Sun sensitivity can also occur, but, according to Mezo, usually not at such a small dose. Tetracycline is not recommended for use with young children, but with nanobacteria this is not usually a consideration because right now the treatment is used primarily in adults.

Misdiagnosing tetracycline allergies. Tetracycline will often cause initial gas, constipation, or stomach upset that subsides after a few days. Moreover, patients sometimes react to the apple juice that is used to mask the taste of the nanobiotic powder, but blame that reaction on the antibiotic. According to Nanobac Pharmaceuticals, and based on some dermatology studies, nanobacteria are also involved in atopic dermatitis, psoriasis, and eczema.[2] When the nanobiotic treatment is started, persons with those disorders may have a mild "Herxheimer reaction" that looks and feels like an allergic reaction, but is not.[3] This is a temporary increase of inflammatory symptoms of a disease when antibiotics are administered.

Suppositories. Americans are not used to putting things up their rectums, because this is not a widely used form of medical application in the United States, except with children and for nausea. Europeans are less queasy because physicians tend to prescribe suppositories more regularly. Not many drugs are administered rectally over four months, so there is some risk that rectal irritation will develop. There is some evidence that irritation of the rectum occurs in lab animals.[4] However, this is also where the issue of relative risk vs. benefits comes into play. If you're 63 years old and dying of heart disease, you're unlikely to worry much about rectal or hemorrhoid irritation. If you're 37, then it may be a consideration to weigh against the risks posed by kidney stones, heart disease, and other ailments.

Unroofing. The treatment can temporarily agitate nanobacteria as they are exposed when their protective coatings are dissolved. Once the fibrotic and fatty layers and thick calcium layers are removed and the nanobacteria are exposed, they get nasty by going from a semi-dormant to suddenly active state. Dr. James Roberts calls this colloquially "pissing them off," causing them to cluster in the blood. That's why it's important to use the right combination of unroofing drugs with the tetracycline that kills them. As pockets of nanobacteria are unroofed, antigen levels go up in patients. This indicates that the nanobacteria have been exposed. If patients do not use the tetracycline or nanobiotic powder, then they may be at risk from clustering of nanobacteria in areas that are constricted by disease. This could trigger further inflammation or clotting. Also, if the treatment is only partially applied, i.e. only some of the ingredients are used, there is a risk of aggravating the infection. Dr. Mezo warns that the absence of a crucial ingredient may be a flaw in other treatments that claim to treat nanobacteria.

A related phenomenon brings up questions about conventional treatments of kidney stones: Do doctors unwittingly unleash nanobacteria by destroying nanobacterial calcified shelters in the form of kidney stones with ultrasound lithotripsy treatments? When a stone is pulverized, it may release billions of nanobacterial particles into our systems, triggering regrowths of calcified deposits that are often recorded. There is as yet minimal evidence to support such a hypothesis, but the discoverers of nanobacteria say that this possibility merits further investigation.

The unknown. The nanobiotic approach has only been prescribed since the year 2000, and although Nanobac Pharmaceuticals says that there have been few reported chronic irritations among the thousands of patients who've taken it, these are still early days. Some doctors say that a few of their patients discontinued the treatment due to a limited tolerance for it. Nonetheless, according to physicians interviewed for this book, indicators of potentially serious trouble, such as reduced kidney or liver function, or increased heart problems, have not yet shown up in tests.[5]

Salvation for the couch potato?

According to Nanobac Pharmaceuticals, this nanobiotic may help to kick-start the body's own abilities to defend itself. In that sense it may improve the basis for good health. Its effectiveness may also be enhanced by exercise and a nutritional diet.

Still, if you think that you can pop a nanobiotic, then be a couch potato, eat badly, drink alcohol heavily, and let your body deteriorate, don't look forward to getting bailed out. The treatment is not a panacea, and patients still need to conduct their lives with due attention to their health.

In patients who are asymptomatic—those who show no clinical signs of illnesses that nanobiotics are designed to treat—the value of preventative application is still unproven. It will take years of testing before it is known whether or to what degree taking the treatment has preventative value. Nonetheless, according to Nanobac Pharmaceuticals, many patients who show few symptoms of illness have enjoyed anecdotal improvements in their general sense of well-being. Mezo points out that not developing atherosclerosis should in theory prevent the onset of other degenerative diseases. Eradicating heavy metal toxicity will decrease the risk of many other diseases. Therefore he says the nanobiotic treatment should have positive effects on general health.

Answering the critics

Criticisms about whether nanobacteria exist or are alive have been described earlier. Other critics have taken aim at the treatment. Their arguments and the response by the treatment's developers can be summarized this way:

1. The treatment is aimed at something that doesn't exist or isn't alive. The existence of something that generates calcification is virtually undisputed, although its classification in biology is yet to be determined. Viruses and prions also fall in the gray zone between being "alive" and being chemical soup ingredients, but they still cause disease. The point is that the treatment targeted at this particular "entity" has been shown to dissolve calcification. Therefore, while the question of how or whether it is alive in conventional terms is important, it does not take away from the fact that the therapy seems to work.

2. There is no evidence that it works. A few years ago it may have been legitimate to claim a lack of clinical evidence about whether or not this treatment reverses heart disease indicators. However, with a growing number of patients showing improved blood work and inflammation indicators, along with later reductions in calcium scores, there are now sufficient results to contest such a claim. Some of these results have been published by qualified cardiologists on the World Wide Web and are available for scrutiny. Prescribing physicians agree that more studies are required and will be done, but they add that early results are promising, and most importantly a treatment is now available, especially for patients who have no other hope.

3. The treatment doesn't meet expectations. There has been disappointment expressed by some prescribing physicians that their patients have not reached the level of decalcification that was originally found in a pilot study by Nanobac Pharmaceuticals.[6] Some patients show no reduction with the first treatment, while others show a substantial reduction. This finding is important, because it points to how the treatment may work. As described earlier, the calcification is often the last thing to go. First, the inflammation and thicker fibrotic cap layers have to be removed. This can take time before other drugs can get at the calcification.

Other mitigating factors include:

✧ Once tissue dies due to total blockage of an artery, the course of treatment requires a more extended timeframe to help microarteries replace the blood flow around the damaged area. Sometimes such regeneration may not occur at all.

✧ Radiologists who do the comparative reading of "before and after" on calcium score removal rates are still gaining experience in how to determine percentages on the CT Scan photographs themselves, especially on older machines. Although the state of the art machines are more accurate and less risky than invasive cardiac catheterization, the overall system is still being optimized.

This has led some critics to say that the reductions in calcium scores being recorded are questionable because they fall within the large margin of error that has been established for reading CT Scan images. Nanobac Pharmaceuticals responds by arguing that the recently completed ACES II cardiology study used newer scanners and software that eliminate much of the error found with older machines.

✧ Researchers also point to a significant accompanying reduction in nanobacterial antigen and antibody levels. These measure the body's response to nanobacteria's presence or absence, and therefore suggest that calcified nanobacteria are being eliminated.

Clinical results show that these antigen and antibody scores often *increase* temporarily as the treatment begins. According to Mezo and as explained earlier, this is because the nanobacteria are being unroofed in massive quantities, and although they are being killed by antibiotics and excreted in urine, their presence in response to nanobacteria can persist for some time after infection, before falling.

4. The treatment is too expensive. The question here is—compared to what? Compare the cost of a nanobacteria treatment—in 2003 this was about $300 USD monthly over four to twelve months—to the cost of open heart surgery, which runs about $25,000 – $50,000. Then add the pain, trouble, lost work days, and risks involved with such surgery, plus the cost of the many drugs that heart patients have to take, running into thousands of dollars per month for the rest of their lives. By contrast, if the nanobacteria treatment continues to be effective after a four to eight month regimen, and patients only require a three or four day per month maintenance treatment after that, then the financial aspects alone—not considering saved pain, hospital visits, and anxiety associated with surgery—represent a savings ratio over heart surgery of about ten to one. In the mid-to-long term, the difference may be far greater.

5. If it's such a great treatment for heart disease, then why does only one company offer it? As described earlier, discovery of nanobacteria and development of a treatment took fifteen years and occurred in the face of substantial skepticism that persists today. Furthermore, methods for detecting and qualifying nanobacteria are still not well known yet. The drug compound is also patent pending. Other companies are already pursuing similar therapies, now that first clinical results are apparent, but they have to acquire the expertise and get around the patent. For example, one clinic is already prescribing tetracycline along with its chelation therapy. Watch for heavy competition in the years ahead. Finally, when wondering why this hasn't taken the world by storm, remember the sad history of the treatment for stomach ulcers...

It's not the first time

The level of skepticism being expressed about the nanobiotic treatment is by no means unusual, nor is it unhealthy as long as it focuses on the scientific burden of proof. But skepticism can often spill over into stubborn resistance in medicine, and that's where the trouble starts.

For those who still ask how such a giant leap might have occurred from looking where so many experts looked before yet found nothing, consider the similar features in the case of stomach ulcers described in Chapter 1.

Helicobacter pylori (the bacteria that causes stomach ulcers) and a treatment for it were discovered many years before they were broadly adopted for treatment of stomach ulcers. In the meantime, thousands of patients had their insides cut out unnecessarily or ineffective drugs prescribed. So, the question relating to nanobacteria is: Will we allow skepticism to spill over into blind resistance, so that a treatment for heart disease experiences the same excruciating delay before it is adopted?

Dr. Stephen Sinatra, a physician who supports the nanobiotic treatment, draws this comparison with the unnecessary stomach surgery that persisted for years:

> In the same way, interventional cardiologists are going in and cutting the blood vessels around patients' hearts to bypass plaque-filled arteries in what has become an alarmingly common procedure. We may learn that all that's needed for severely calcified arteries is a course of the right antibiotic.[7]

CHAPTER TWELVE

Who Pays As The Patient Revolution Unfolds?

After years of medical choices being governed by Health Maintenance Organizations (HMOs) in America, it is clear that the "managed care" experiment isn't working. Exasperated physicians, patients, and insurers agree that the "healthcare" system has become a "sickness care" system that is broken and broke. Although HMOs are often blamed, many factors have added to the debacle:

- ✧ The population is getting older and, as it does, health problems and costs increase.

- ✧ Western medicine's emphasis on treating instead of preventing disease has proven horrendously expensive as epidemics such as obesity and heart disease grow. Treatments that mask symptoms do not cure disease, so the problems get worse.

- ✧ Fraud, government regulation, and pressure from drug and medical equipment company shareholders to deliver profits have worsened the price spiral.

✧ While costs skyrocket, patients don't get the care that they want and doctors can't give patients the care that they think they need because insurers often won't pay for it and patients often can't afford it themselves.

✧ Patients and doctors are fed up being told by third parties what treatments they can get or prescribe. As a consequence, insurers find themselves being sued for decisions to withhold treatments from, or dictate them to, patients.

These may seem like generalizations, but a look at healthcare costs testifies to the problem. In the year 2000, those costs increased more than eight percent—about four times more than the inflation rate—to constitute fourteen percent of America's gross domestic product. Health insurance premiums for employers and employees grew by about thirteen percent in 2002 then continued along similar lines in 2003.[1]

Those were not exceptions. They reflected a trend of the past decade. Many of the increases were for heart disease treatment.

It is therefore important to see how nanobiotics might fit into the cost picture. This requires knowing what is being tried to control runaway medical expenses.

How it began

Dr. Alan Iezzi, M.D., F.A.A.F.P. is a practicing physician, but also co-founder and medical director of Patient Directed Care, one of a few companies that broke away from managed care by letting members have unimpeded access to healthcare at a discounted rate, without going through an insurer.[2]

Iezzi gives his view of how and why the managed care system got America into such a predicament:

"The original idea for insurance was that you pay a small premium to cover the back-end expense. Today you're paying a high premium and covering most of the expense. *The real question is, are [patients] really buying insurance today?* Insurance today has a high deductible. I see ranges from five hundred to five thousand dollars per annum. That's enough to cover most medical procedures."[3]

Deductibles hurt especially young families and the elderly. Iezzi says that most younger patients spend less than a thousand or two thousand dollars in medical expenses in any one year. Yet their deductibles are often more than that, so insurance is useless. Their premiums are also much more than three or four years ago. Most employers are unable or unwilling to pay for such increases. Meanwhile, government Medicaid and Medicare programs are jacking up deductibles for the elderly.

These cost pressures have led many patients to take matters into their own hands. For years now, busloads of seniors have been crossing the U.S. border into Canada to get the same drugs at much lower cost. Many of these are heart disease drugs. This trickle has become a flood since Canadian companies began selling those drugs via mail order. The pharmaceuticals industry has responded by lobbying legislators to ban such imports, but local and state governments that carry the brunt of the load for funding seniors healthcare are balking at such a ban because it cuts into their overloaded budgets. The argument has erupted into an intergovernmental brawl, with patients stuck in between.[4]

Contributing to the rise in deductibles and premiums has been a low interest rate policy of the past few years that has hurt insurers' ability to make profits from non-medical financial transactions.

"Insurers are looking to make a higher profit in an investment environment that doesn't allow them to make money on investments and to pay dividends to shareholders," Iezzi says. "So they're having to raise premiums. The cost of that is being passed to the employee."[5]

Many legislators and patients blame the cost increase on malpractice suits, but studies show such blame to be misplaced. The same phenomenon of low investment returns for insurers is the prime culprit in driving up doctors' malpractice insurance premiums. Therefore, patients' rights groups argue that putting a cap on malpractice settlements as some legislatures have done will not lower malpractice premiums or bring savings to patients.[6]

Then there is the middleman.

"The difference between healthcare in the [nineteen] forties and now is that most healthcare was paid for directly by the patient to the doctor, and the decisions were made by the patient and the physician. Today healthcare is delivered by physicians to patients, but is mediated by third parties.

"It evolved to provide post World War II Americans with security from catastrophic illness that might come from, [for example], nuclear fallout. We're the post-bomb generation, so there is fear in the unknown. Hence the insurance industry took over to provide a system that would work in the event that catastrophic illness would prevail. Since then, that simple approach has become a very large industry that took it upon themselves (sic) to be the mediator of healthcare.

"It wasn't just the bomb exploding but also technology exploding. Post-World War II technology exploded as well as [the development of] diagnostic equipment—better X-ray equipment, CAT scans. The practice of medicine has always been to provide better diagnostic tools for patients.

"The other thing," Iezzi adds, "is that procedures and testing are more expensive. So as costs mounted, the industry started to look at how to mitigate the costs because they were writing bigger checks than they were taking in as premiums. So they said, 'Well, you can't use this technology. We haven't evaluated its accuracy or its use in a particular disease.' So physicians—who are also scientists—for the first time were not able to provide the use of current and up-to-date technology to best determine what their patients might need.

"Today you have very informed patients who are very well read on current technologies and their use. But you have insurers in the middle who say, 'we are not going to approve that.'

"What *doesn't* happen is that patients say 'Well, I'm going to pay for that out of my pocket', so it doesn't get done. That carries over into prescription writing and into treatments.

"Use the coronary artery as an example: You diagnose it with Ultra-fast CAT scanning. But [most] insurers today don't approve that because it has not been brought into their realm as a treatment.

"So you have this system in the middle that prevents patients from getting state of the art care."[7]

The gradual shift to prevention

As the patient and physician backlash compounds cost woes for insurers, HMOs have begun to pay for preventative health visits. Iezzi characterizes this as the difference between "indemnity" that only pays for illness, and "preventative health maintenance" where patients come in healthier and earlier.

Preventative health maintenance makes sense, Iezzi says, because it reduces disabilities and hospitalizations, while increasing working life via healthy longevity.

Still, he says, the same problem remains: Physicians are limited in what they can use for diagnosing or treating diseases because often the tools aren't covered by insurers.

One example he cites is the PSA test (Prostate Specific Antigen blood test), now the gold standard for diagnosing prostate cancer. For years it was not covered by most health maintenance organizations because it was not apparently proven effective, "whereas in the literature," he explains, "it was obvious that it was a viable way to check for prostate cancer." Unfortunately, it was also expensive.

Similarly, with heart disease, Dr. Iezzi says, "Hospitalization and results of end stage disease are the big costs for the insurance industry. So why not pay $300 for a coronary artery scan (as a preventative measure) rather than spend $2,000 on catheterization?"

Self-directed plans

In response to this, some employers and insurers are finally beginning to pay for patients to manage their own preventative healthcare via savings and discount systems that minimize red tape.

One concept is based roughly on the federal government's Medical Savings Accounts that give spending discretion to employees.

Just like self-directed pension plans, this aims to shift responsibility to workers. The advantage is that it gives the individual more freedom to choose. The tough part is that workers have to be more sophisticated in their approach to healthcare services.

The plans work like this: The employer provides every employee with a tax-free healthcare fund of $1,000 - $2,000 annually. That doesn't sound like much, but as explained earlier, most younger individuals spend less than that annually on healthcare.[8] For older heart patients this is also close to what a course of nanobiotic therapy costs.

The surprise of dealing with catastrophic illness is the exception to such regular medical expenditures, but there is usually separate lower-cost insurance for this less likely scenario among the young.

With self-directed plans, the employee can use the money for medical services that they want. They can choose their own doctors, get an eye exam, or go for alternative treatment. In such plans there is no "co-pay" where an insurer that shares expenses has to approve them; no bureaucrats making medical decisions for patients, and just as importantly, no red tape for getting your money back. If funds are left at year-end, the employee can sometimes, but not always, roll them over into next year.

The growth in these plans may account for much of the rapid increase in workers researching health providers more carefully. It may also explain at least part of the dramatic rise in alternative health services being offered by reputable hospitals across America.

Who is providing the insurance plans? One of the first is Definity Health, based in Minneapolis, that has offered them since about 1999. Others include Aetna, Humana Inc., Destiny Health, First Health Group Corp. and Wellpoint Health Networks Inc.'s Unicare Health Plans of Illinois.[9]

Are companies using the plans for their employees? So far a small minority of corporations have offered them, but the schemes seem to be growing in popularity.

One outcome is that many hospitals have started preventative care clinics that cater to demands for other types of health services.[10] The depth of this revolution is only now becoming apparent in America, while it has been going on for some time in Europe and Asia.

Nanobiotics and prevention

An early indicator of this wave is that some insurers have opted to pay for the nanobiotic treatment. While researchers argue over what nanobacteria are and in what category they fit, some doctors find the treatment effective and less expensive than traditional therapies. Insurers are supporting such decisions.

This is the opposite of how things normally happen in insurance.

The procedure used to work like this: It had to be proven beyond a reasonable doubt that something was causing a disease. Then, after exhaustive trials, proof had to be given that symptoms could be treated with a specific regimen. Then and only then, the insurance industry might have looked at it.

Not anymore. Especially for seriously ill patients where conventional approaches have been exhausted, the process is being re-engineered because insurers, employers and patients are looking for cost-effective solutions that aim at a cause instead of a symptom.

Discounted medical services

The problem with medical savings plans described earlier is that they provide limited funds. There is a resulting risk that patients will put off treatment to save money. This is especially true with older patients who may delay treatments that exceed the cost limit of such plans.

For this group, but also for young families who balk at spiralling deductibles in their conventional insurance, another approach is being tried.

Patient Directed Care is one of a few companies that is embarking on what may be the next big approach to healthcare. Alan Iezzi says that the company's strategy has been to start with the principle that patients need to direct—and pay directly for—their own care, but not without help.

In this case, the insurance company has been cut out of the patient-physician relationship.

"We've eliminated the whole insurance middleman," he says. Patients "can go to anyone who's agreed to provide the discount. They pay directly, there's no claims filing."

His company contracts with healthcare providers to provide discounts to members of the plan. The patient signs up and has access to the network at a prearranged price. The discount is equal to what the managed care plans pay to the physicians right now, but the paperwork has been slashed.

The patient is given something like a debit card, that lets them pay for services on the spot. The discount runs up to 60-70 percent. According to Iezzi, much of that—up to thirty percentage points—is generated from less paperwork by cutting out the insurance company.

Due to those reduced costs, most healthcare providers also get paid more than what they'd get by going through the insurer, so it's attractive to them as well.

Moreover says Iezzi, ninety percent of this type of care is delivered outside the hospitals, reducing strain on those systems while saving patients the discomfort of long hospital waiting room visits.

Part of that new patient-directed approach is made possible by the Internet, where patients can go to a website and get their test results quickly.

How to pay for nanobiotics?

Likewise, he adds, since nanobiotics are a viable option for treating and reversing coronary artery disease, it makes sense for this plan to encourage their use.

Iezzi first heard about nanobiotics from Drs. Mezo and Maniscalco. It was Maniscalco's guarded enthusiasm about the results that caused him to examine nanobacteria more closely.

Iezzi was looking at this from the viewpoint of its potential impacts on healthcare delivery—how the treatment might help to make healthcare more patient-directed than the third party system that is in place now.

He says that screening for nanobacteria will be offered in the same way. The company hopes to recommend the NanobacTEST-S for blood and NanobacTEST-U/A for urine on their website to a certain type of patient who might benefit from such a preventative diagnostic tool. That patient would then go to any authorized lab, get the test done, then go to their own passworded file on the website and see the results. The whole process happens without going to an insurer or hospital.

Will patient-directed discounts fly? Several companies are betting on it.

Advanced PCS (http://www.advancepcsrx.com)
Aetna Inc. (http://www.aetna.com)
Anthem Blue Cross/ Blue Shield (http://www.anthem.com)
Blue Cross/Blue Shield Florida (http://bcbsfl.com)
Blue Cross/Blue Shield of Rhode Island (http://www.bcbsri.com)
Blue Cross/Blue Shield of West Michigan (http://www.bcbsmi.com)
Capital Blue Cross/Blue Shield (http://www.bcbs.com)
Caremark (http://www.caremark.com)
Central Reserve Life (http://www.centralreserve.com)
Cigna (http://www.cigna.com)
Emerald Health (http://www.emeraldhealth.com)
Express Scripts (http://www.express-scripts.com)
Humana (http://www.humana.com)
Mail Handlers (http://www.firsthealth.com)
Medco (http://www.medcohealth.com)
National Association of Letter Carriers   (http://www.nalc.com)
Pacific Source Health (http://www.pacificsource.com)
Tricare/ Tricare for Life (http://www.tricare.osd.mil)
United Health Care Insurance Company (http://www.unitedhealthcare.com)
Walgreens Health Initiatives (http://www.whphi.com)
Note: This list is not comprehensive. Some of these companies give only partial reimbursement based on the treatment being a compounded medication, and according to the patient's policy terms. Most companies that have a provision in their policies for compounded drugs will probably reimburse.]

Figure 10: Insurers that may cover nanobiotics

Meanwhile a few conventional insurers are already reimbursing patients for NanobacTX. Figure 10 shows insurers that may cover the nanobiotic treatment.[11] Many of these insurers make decisions whether to pay for treatment at the local level on a case by case basis. It often depends on whether a policy covers compounded medications. Therefore just because they pay in one region for one patient does not guarantee that they will pay in every case as a company-wide policy.

Nanobiotics have also become a more viable consideration for elderly patients, because as Medicaid deductibles rise, they find themselves hit with a big monthly bill for heart drugs that they have been told they must take for the rest of their lives. This is inspiring many to look for treatments that deal with the underlying problem instead of just the symptoms. Nanobiotics are among the few if not the only ones to do this in heart disease. By helping to minimize the need for surgery and other drugs, they may give seniors a way to cut costs of the coronary merry-go-round that many stay stuck on forever.

Healing the homeless with nanobiotics?

The systems described here may work well for health-savvy patients, but what about one of the most expensive problems in healthcare? This is commonly referred to as "indigent medical care," or treating the homeless and working poor.

There are about twenty thousand "indigent" individuals in Hillsborough county, Florida, where Dr. Iezzi works. These are the truly homeless, and also those who have a job but after basic amenities don't have anything left to pay for insurance or medical care.

Iezzi explains that every county in the U.S. has the obligation to care for its indigent population, and every county has a different way of doing that. Traditionally hospitals take on most of the load for delivering care to indigent persons, who often use the emergency room to get services. In the past that was billed back to the federal and state governments. But that system ended after the federal government abandoned reimbursement for homeless healthcare. Now, says Iezzi, "either the hospital does it as goodwill or the county contracts with doctors at very low rates and that is taxed to the taxpayers."

That's exactly what happens in Hillsborough County, which includes most of Tampa, where a portion of the sales tax goes to fund indigent care. That sales tax was so unpopular that it was once reduced. Yet when funds ran out, the tax had to be raised again. Despite an innovative cost-cutting approach that delivers care in a coordinated way and has won national recognition, Hillsborough County still faces a big bill. "That's ninety million dollars a year," says Iezzi. "It's huge."[12]

The trend is seen in most American counties. Federal government abandonment of support for indigent healthcare is forcing local governments to take it on. To make matters worse, they are legislatively prohibited from running deficits, so the money has to come from current revenues.

Looking at this, it becomes clear why preventative treatments are growing attractive to local governments, compared to costly "end-of-pipe" heart disease therapies that address the symptoms instead of the cause.

While the preventive approach is being considered by governments and insurers, privatization of indigent healthcare is also being tried by some counties to cut costs. Unfortunately, says Iezzi, experience shows that privatization alone doesn't solve the problem. It can make it worse if private systems fail and patients end up at hospitals.

Another large group falls just outside the category of "indigent"; those who are below the poverty line but not in the legal category of poor. They too head to the hospital emergency room for their needs.

Thus, Iezzi maintains that a preventative healthcare approach is required to make privatization work. Otherwise, the hospital emergency systems will break down as before.

Few physicians argue against such a preventative maintenance approach. Yet to be effective it must have cardiovascular disease high on the list of pre-emptive targets. The nanobiotic drug treatment might fit the bill as part of an affordable preventative strategy that insurers and state agencies can support.

Right now the main beneficiaries of the treatment are patients who already have the disease. That too helps insurers by slashing hospitalization costs. But it also suggests that more research is required to determine the effectiveness in patients who have just early symptoms.

This takes us back to the question of what we know and what we don't about a "cure" for heart disease.

CHAPTER THIRTEEN

What We Know And What We Don't

Until recently, the reply to "*Has heart disease been cured?*" was a resounding *No.* But now we have learned that the reply has changed to a hopeful *Maybe* for the widespread illness known as atherosclerosis.

Clinical results suggest that the deadliest factors in this disease—inflammation, clotting, and arterial plaque—are not only being controlled; they are also being reversed. That may not be a "cure" yet, but it seems that something has been found to gradually get rid of a trigger for coronary artery and vascular disease.

We know further that hundreds if not thousands of patients who might have otherwise paid handsomely for surgery have so far avoided it and saved themselves, their insurers, and the economy a financial hit.

If we go back to the beginning of this book and ask, "*What does it mean to be cured?*" we see that many villains including inflammation, soft and hard calcified plaque, and harmful clotting have to be convincingly dealt with, then kept at bay. According to the physicians who prescribe it, the nanobiotic treatment described in this book deals effectively with many of these culprits.

However, then the patient has to be restored to health.

Because it has a therapeutic history of only a few years and is used primarily with patients who are so sick that they have major accumulated damage, it is hard to say if it qualifies as a "cure." As explained earlier, someone who has suffered the ravages of leprosy and who is then "cured" still has scars that may lead to a shortened life. The same rule may apply to damage left by coronary heart disease, although we don't know for sure because we don't have sufficient experience with reversing it.

Certainly more work is required with patients where the condition is less advanced. This means working with more patients who are in their thirties, forties, and fifties.

Nonetheless, if early results from the nanobiotic treatment hold true, they may transform the way that heart medicine is practiced by confirming the emerging unifying theory of atherogenesis that has been largely developed by Gary Mezo, Olavi Kajander, Neva Çiftçioglu, and their many collaborators.

At the core of that work are calcium and a nanoscale factory—*Nanobacterium sanguineum*—that uses it. Calcium is the stuff of life and death. It is everywhere in our bodies and we wouldn't be here without it. Yet it also kills us when processes that utilize it go haywire. We know more about why we calcify than we did only a few years ago. We know, although some contest the idea, that entities named nanobacteria generate "apatite" and that the resulting calcified deposits cause trouble throughout the body. We know how to get rid of them with nanobiotics. The first of these is a product known as NanobacTX. There is preliminary evidence that we might be able to use it to treat many of the diseases—from kidney stones to cataracts—where calcification has been shown to be present.

Still, what we don't know far exceeds what we do. How do nanobacteria mineralize and what is their precise role in kidney stone and other calcification related diseases? Does their eradication prevent stone formation?

The structure of nanobacteria that initiates calcification remains imprecisely defined, as does their potential role in cancer and many other diseases. We don't know the final details of their DNA and RNA although we have seen many parts of these genetic building blocks. It is surprising, for example, that more than fifteen years after *Nanobacterium sanguineum* was discovered and ten years after nanobacterium was patented, no major research institution has yet published investigations into its DNA structure, or announced that it has tried to ascertain its contents with new methods such as Atomic Force Microscopy or Scanning Tunneling Microscopy. It seems that ongoing skepticism about whether nanobacteria exist, despite convincing evidence to the contrary, is still preventing such work, although one would think that this would spur researchers to prove or disprove the organisms' characteristics.

In this respect, we know that medical authorities have sometimes been slow to acknowledge infection in disease, as was the case with stomach ulcers. Hopefully, lessons have been learned from that experience. Skepticism is not a justification for obstruction.

We know some of the ways in which nanobacteria enter cells, but we don't know others. We don't know how long they can live, but it seems years or perhaps far longer, especially in their dormant state.

Might nanobacteria cause osteoporosis—loss of bone density—in so many women by interfering with the normal calcium exchanges in the body? What role might they play in fetal heart abnormalities associated with calcification? What about the many other diseases described in this book that involve calcification?

Once we get rid of the initial nanobacterial infection, can we keep it at bay forever? Will nanobacteria develop resistance to the treatment? Are there other drugs that might be more effective than NanobacTX? Why do some patients get better faster than others? Are some persons immune to nanobacteria?

Might some nanobacteria be good for us? There is no evidence of that yet, but if they are so prevalent in our environment, who knows? The underlying mysteries remain: Where did they come from, how old are they, and what form of life are they truly? Were they used by nature millions of years ago to store valuable calcium and phosphate that are essential ingredients for cell life? Are they still used for such a purpose?

Then there is the issue of other infections. So many bacteria and viruses—including *Herpes*, *Chlamydia*, and dental germs—have been found in atherosclerosis.[1] Are they secondary to nanobacteria infections, or do they somehow interact with them at the beginning?

Much more research is required to find the answers to these questions. Much is underway. By the time this book is published, some of that research will be completed. To keep up with such research and controversy, continuous updates will be made to a website relating to this work and to other editions of this book.[2]

Despite the elementary state of our knowledge, important discoveries have been made. There are now tests to detect the presence of entities that trigger inflammation and calcification in the vascular and urinary systems. There is a treatment that according to statistical analysis reverses clinical markers of atherosclerosis. These methods are available to millions who might otherwise die or suffer unnecessarily, and to millions more among their families and friends who face the financial and psychological burdens of heart disease.

That is what we know.

Milestones

Here are highlights of the research into nanoscale life forms and a trigger for pathological calcification. The term "announces," when used below, signifies that the date shown was the year of publication. If that term is not used, then the date denotes the year when the discovery was reported to have occurred, but may not have been published in a journal at that time.

1985   Olavi Kajander observes nanoscale particles *in vitro*, forming a community, as contaminants in mammalian cell cultures. He surmises that they may be alive. Labs fail to grow them due to the particles' special properties.

1986   Robert Folk observes nanoscale entities in geological formations, but he does not publish findings for years.[1]

1986/87   Kajander observes that some of the particles he found earlier seem to have a hard surface.

1987   Kajander discovers the particles in human blood.

1988   Kajander takes first electron microscope pictures of them and develops polyclonal antibodies to detect them.

1990   Kajander files for patent for nanobacteria, plus culturing and antibody methods.

1991   Neva Çiftçioglu and Kajander develop new monoclonal antibodies to detect nanobacteria.

1992   Kajander is awarded a patent for nanobacteria and related detection methods.[2]

1992   Çiftçioglu discovers that nanobacteria make mineralized "igloo-like" structures. These explained the hard surfaces observed earlier.

1992   Kajander et al. publish one of the first abstracts on blood nanobacteria.[3]

1992   Çiftçioglu and Kajander develop medium that makes nanobacteria grow quickly.

1993   Optimized methods for detecting nanobacteria antigen are developed by Kajander and his company as a prototype for the commercial methods used today.

1996   David McKay et al. announce discovery of nanoscale organisms in a meteorite.[4] A controversy over nanobacteria begins.

1996   Kajander, Çiftçioglu et al. announce discovery of potential nanobacteria contamination in antibody products.[5]

1997   Akerman, Kuikka, Çiftçioglu, Parkkinen, Bergstrom, Kuronen, and Kajander announce discovery that nanobacteria replicate in rabbits, fulfilling part of Koch's postulate.[6]

1998   Gary Mezo develops a compounded prescription drug to treat heart disease and administers it to four heart patients with encouraging results. Then he applies to patent it. He also begins to conduct a pilot study of other patients.

1998   Çiftçioglu and Kajander announce discoveries that EDTA unroofs nanobacteria and that tetracycline kills them.

1998   Çiftçioglu and Kajander announce discovery of nanobacteria in kidney stones.[7] The story is covered by journals and news services worldwide.

1998   N. Çiftçioglu, V. Çiftçioglu, H. Vali, E. Turcott, and O. Kajander announce discovery of nanobacteria in dental stones.[8]

1998   Philippa J. R. Uwins *et al.* announce discovery of nano-organisms ("nanobes") in Australian sandstone. This receives media coverage.

1999   László Puskás, who met Kajander and Çiftçioglu in 1996, detects nanobacteria in atherosclerotic plaque and submits to journals but cannot get findings published.

1999   The Finnish start-up company Nanobac Oy begins using tests for diagnosing nanobacteria in patients with heart and kidney disease.

1999-   Charges against Kajander that his investigations
2000   into nanobacteria were fraudulent are officially investigated and dismissed as groundless.

2000   Garcia-Cuerpo *et al.* fulfill Koch's postulates for proving nanobacteria as infectious agents.[9]

2000   Thomas Hjelle, Marcia Miller-Hjelle, Çiftçioglu *et al.* announce discovery of nanobacteria in Polycystic Kidney Disease.[10]

2000   Mezo meets Kajander and Çiftçioglu, then adds tetracycline to his prescription treatment to kill nanobacteria.

2001   Çiftçioglu and Kajander announce detection of nanobacteria in viral vaccines as reported by *Vaccines Today* and *New Scientist*.[11]

2001   First Nanobacteria Symposium is held in Kuopio Finland to bring principal nanobacteria researchers together.

2002   NanobacLabs (now Nanobac Pharmaceuticals) license Nanobac Oy laboratory tests for detecting nanobacteria.

2002   Karl Stetter *et al.* announce discovery of nanoarchaeae in volcanic vents and sequence the organism's DNA.

2002   American cardiologists begin to report that their patients have sustained reductions in heart disease markers after treatment with NanobacTX developed by Gary Mezo.

2002   Rasmussen *et al.* duplicate László Puskás work, finding nanobacteria in atherosclerotic plaque.[12]

2002   Çiftçioglu and Kajander announce discovery of contamination of gamma globulin products with nanobacteria.[13]

2002   Mezo, Benedict Maniscalco *et al.* initiate first formal independent clinical trial of NanobacTX.

2003   Martin Kerner *et al.* announce discovery of nanoscale entities that replicate in bacteria-like ways in polluted river water.[14]

2003   First clinical trial of NanobacTX completed. Maniscalco announces preliminary significant reductions in calcium scores and other markers of atherosclerosis.[15]

2003   Kajander, Maniscalco, Aho, and Mezo put forward unified theory of atherogenesis and treatment based on nanobacteria.[16]

Fulfilling Koch's Postulates

The ground rules observed by every medical scientist for proving the relationship between an organism and disease are known as Koch's postulates, developed by physician and bacteriologist Robert Koch around the turn of the 20th century. The postulates hold that these conditions must be fulfilled:

1. The microorganism must be detectable in the infected host at every stage of the disease.

2. The microorganism must be isolated from the diseased host and grown in pure culture.

3. When susceptible, healthy animals are infected with pathogens from the pure culture, the specific symptoms of the disease must occur.

4. The microorganism must be re-isolated from the diseased animal and correspond to the original microorganism in pure culture.

In 2000 and 2001, Garcia-Cuerpo *et al.* published research papers in the Spanish Journal of Urology[17] outlining how they had met each condition by injecting nanobacteria into healthy laboratory animals, then tracing them through the metabolism, finding them in excreted urine, detecting them in kidney damage, and culturing the extracted nanobacteria from resulting kidney stone samples.

[Note: As with the rest of this book, the Milestones list is copyrighted by the authors and permission must be obtained prior to copying or distributing it in whole or in part.]

Acknowledgements

This book would not have been possible without the on-going co-operation of (in alphabetical order) Neva Çiftçioglu, Olavi Kajander, and Gary Mezo. The insights they gave into their pioneering work on nanobacteria were invaluable.

A special note of appreciation goes to Gary Mezo for putting us in contact with so many of the major players, for accepting our "warts and all" approach to this topic, and for his extensive discussions on wide-ranging matters. The staff of Nanobac Pharmaceuticals, although they shall remain unnamed at the request of the company, also provided helpful insights into the advantages and drawbacks of the present NanobacTX therapy along with the tests for detecting nanobacteria.

The authors are indebted to Benedict Maniscalco, who let us witness some often-blunt discussions about what has to be done to optimize a treatment for controlling atherosclerosis.

Among the physicians who have been prescribing the nanobiotic treatment, James C. Roberts gave us keen insights into his experiences, especially with EECP and EDTA related therapies. Appreciation goes to Alan Iezzi for his special insight into the medical insurance industry.

To the other medical reviewers who consented to check this text: Thank you. Also, to the Association for

Eradication of Heart Attack (AEHA) for their illustrations of atherosclerosis.

To our friends, siblings, and colleagues who critiqued our work, it was appreciated.

To The Writers' Collective, who are pioneering a new way of publishing that gives authors more control over their work.

Most of all thanks to the patients who let us into parts of their private lives normally reserved for the physician-patient relationship: We hope that this book justifies the trust that you've put in us so that others may benefit.

APPENDICES

Plain Language Glossary

This glossary is for non-medical readers who want to understand technical terms used in this book. The explanations are not just borrowed from medical dictionaries, but instead have been customized to explain terms as they relate to calcification and nanobacteria. There is, to our knowledge, no other glossary that explains such terms in this context.

Anecdotal evidence – Findings that are based on casual observations or indications rather than rigorous or scientific analysis. "I feel better," or "My pain seemed to go away" are anecdotal statements. Clinical evidence does not depend on such anecdotal reports. In this book, observations of patients who have taken treatments for nanobacterial infections are divided into anecdotal and clinical evidence. See "clinical evidence."

Aneurysm – A dangerous blood-filled dilation of a blood vessel caused by disease or weakening of the vessel's wall. This can cut off blood supply and cause death. Researchers theorize that aneurysms can be caused by calcification and by nanobacterial infections.

Angina – Chest pain and feeling of tightness brought on by reduced oxygen supply to the heart, often associated with partial blockage of the coronary arteries by calcified deposits.

Angiogram – An X-ray of blood vessels that shows obstructions in the vessels when the patient receives an injection of dye to outline the vessels on the X-ray. This is generally regarded as being more accurate but more risky than a CT scan and less accurate than catheterization when an instrument is inserted directly into the vessel. The accuracy with which angiograms can show inflammation and calcification is questionable because inflammation can vary in patients from time to time, and some calcium deposits won't show up on the angiogram. See also CT scan.

Angioplasty – Widening of a partially or fully blocked artery by inserting a hollow wire that is then inflated. Angioplasties often reblock over months or years. It is theorized that the procedure may release large amounts of nanobacteria that trigger the reblocking process.

Ankylosing Spondylitis – Chronic inflammation of vertebrae in the spine. It can immobilize a patient. Calcification is found in this condition.

Antibodies – Cells that are purpose-built by the immune system to deal with infections that enter the body. Because of their ability to precisely "recognize" and bind to certain shapes on other molecules, antibody binding is also used by researchers to identify organisms. In the case of nanobacteria, antibodies have been engineered to test for their presence.

Antigens – Substances that cause an immune reaction in the body. A bacteria, virus, or other pathogen can be an antigen. These are also used as markers to identify the presence of infections such as nanobacteria.

Apatite (Hydroxyl Apatite) – Calcium phosphate mineral found in rocks, bone, teeth, kidney stones, and atherosclerosis. Not to be confused with calcium carbonate, which is another type of deposit.

Atherosclerosis – A form of heart disease characterized by the deposition of plaques containing cholesterol and lipids on the innermost layer of the walls of large and medium-sized arteries. Calcification and nanobacteria have frequently been found in atherosclerosis. Nanobacteria seem to trigger it. It is one of several types of "Arteriosclerosis," a disease characterized by thickening and hardening of artery walls.

Atopic Dermatitis – Inflammation of the skin resulting from a hereditary predisposition to developing hypersensitivity reactions. Calcification is associated with this condition.

Calcification (Pathological) – Deposition of calcium compounds in parts of the body where they are not supposed to be, producing harmful results consistent with the pathogenic behavior of an organism. Here are a few related terms used by your physician to describe calcification in the body:

Apatite (not appetite), brain sand (calcium deposits in the brain), calcified cysts, calcified deposits, calcinosis, calcium deposition and buildup, calcium phosphate ($CaPO_4$), dystrophic calcification (results from disease at the site of calcification), extraskeletal calcification (calcification that takes place outside your skeleton), hard plaque, hardening, metastatic calcification (results from disease remote from the site of calcification that has caused elevated blood calcium or phosphate), microcalcification (often found in breast cancer), ossification, plaque, spurs, and stones.

Calcium score – A calculation that shows the buildup of calcium salts in the arteries. This is done, for example, with Electron Beam Computed Tomography (EBCT). It is used to identify apparently healthy individuals who are at high risk of heart attack, but who do not fit the usual profile with risk factors such as obesity and smoking. Calcium scores can range from zero to more than three thousand. Zero is often good. Three thousand is not. Calcium scoring is still an inexact science in terms of precisely comparing scores in one individual over time, but new technology has improved accuracy greatly in the past few years. Although calcium scores have been identified as good predictors of cardiovascular disease, there is no apparent correlation between fitness and high or low calcium scores.[1] This seems to run contrary to conventional wisdom about how to ward off a heart attack. One would think that a "fit" person should have a lower calcium score, because such persons are supposed to be at less risk of heart disease. Yet this is often not the case. When we consider that many who suffer heart attacks have had no prior symptoms and are often consider "fit," then the calcium scores start to make more sense. Someone who is in great shape but who has a high calcium score is at risk of heart disease. Until calcium scoring was developed, we didn't know this.

Cardiac catheterization – Inserting a tube into the arteries to check for blockage.

Chelation therapy – A treatment to remove heavy metals from the blood. Commonly used for lead poisoning. The most common form is intravenous chelation where a solution containing chelating agents such as the chemical EDTA is injected into the body along with mineral supplements to balance the effects on the body. The chemical binds with heavy metals. Then the combination is excreted in urine.

Cholesterol –

> **Good** HDL, or high-density lipoproteins, are often referred to as "good cholesterol." HDL carries cholesterol from your tissues and returns it to the liver. It is called "good" because higher levels of HDL allegedly reduces your risk of developing cardiovascular disease.

> **Bad** LDL, or low-density lipoproteins, carry the cholesterol from the liver to the other tissues. It is called "bad" because higher levels of LDL allegedly increase your risk of developing cardiovascular diseases.

> **Indifferent** Some physicians argue that cholesterol does not cause heart disease and is not a reliable predictor of who may have a heart attack.[2]

Clinical evidence – Something that is based on direct observation of a patient by a qualified physician. Clinical diagnosis, study, trial, and proof are each predicated on such observations. For example, clinical evidence of changes in a heart patient's condition includes measurements of blood pressure, stress, pulse, "good" and "bad" cholesterol, triglycerides, calcification, inflammation indicators such as C-reactive protein, erythrocyte sedimentation rate, fibrinogen, and white blood cell count. These are fundamental to understanding whether a treatment aimed at nanobacterial infection also has impacts on heart disease. They are also fundamentally different from anecdotal evidence, which is far less measurable.

CRP C-reactive protein – An indicator of inflammation that is used to predict heart attack risk in healthy adults. Since the role of inflammation in heart disease is crucial, the role of CRP is becoming increasingly important as a measure of that inflammation. According to an article published by the American Heart Association, although CRP is a good predictor, it is not yet known if lowering CRP levels alone reduces the risk of cardiovascular disease.[3]

CT Scan – Cardiac Tomography – Form of X-ray used to provide cross-sectional images of the chest, including the heart and great vessels. It can be used to show calcification but is considered an older technology. For newer technology, see Electron Beam Computed Tomography.

Diabetes – A disorder characterized by excessive urination and thirst. It is often associated with heart disease. Overweight individuals are subject to becoming diabetic. Calcification is often associated with advanced diabetes.

DNA – Deoxyribonucleic Acid – Considered to be one of the building blocks of life and a basis for genetic science. A nucleic acid carries the genetic information in the cell and is capable of self-replication. Bacteria and nanobacteria each have DNA, but this does not make them the same life forms.

EDTA – EDTA is a colorless organic compound used to bind and extract heavy metals. It is the preferred treatment for lead poisoning and has been used for this over more than fifty years. The term chelation stems from the Greek word "chele," meaning claw, as EDTA chemically grabs metal particles (such as aluminum, lead, mercury, and cadmium) and minerals (such as calcium) like a claw. Once in the blood stream, it binds to these elements. The resulting combination of EDTA, metals, and minerals is excreted from the body during urination.

EECP – Enhanced External Counter Pulsation – A procedure where pneumatic cuffs are placed over the patient's lower extremity, then inflated and deflated repeatedly. This drives oxygenated blood backwards from the lower parts of the body into the heart. That in turn increases pressure between the open arteries and those that are blocked by heart disease. This pressure stimulates formation of small natural "bypasses."

Electron Beam Computed Tomography (EBCT) – A fast form of X-ray imaging technology. Also known as an Ultrafast

CT Scan. An EBCT scan takes about 90 seconds and detects calcium deposits associated with heart disease and other ailments.[4] It can take multiple images of the heart within the time of a single heartbeat, providing details about the heart's function and structures and slashing the time required for a study.

Endotoxin – A toxin produced by bacteria and by nanobacteria that is toxic to other cells and often elicits an immune reaction by the body.

Fetal bovine serum (FBS) – Extract from baby cow blood used to develop vaccines and grow cells for experiments. The serum has been found to be contaminated with nanobacteria.

Fibrinogen – A protein in the blood plasma that is essential for the coagulation or thickening of blood. It is one of the indicators of heart disease. It is used by the body to close off injured blood vessel walls. Elevated levels suggest that the atherosclerotic process is occurring.[5]

HDL – See Cholesterol.

Herxheimer Reaction – Nicknamed "herx" after Jarisch-Herxheimer, it is a temporary increase of symptoms of a disease when some drugs are administered. It can seem like an allergic reaction to an antibiotic, but it is not.

High blood pressure - Hypertension – Blood pressure is the force of blood against the walls of arteries. Blood pressure rises and falls during the day. When it stays elevated over time, it is called high blood pressure or hypertension. This is considered a measure of stroke or heart attack risk.[6]

In vitro – An artificial environment outside the body, such as a test tube or petri dish. Many biological experiments, such as culturing bacteria, are done *in vitro,* as opposed to *in vivo* (inside the body).

Inflammation – A normally healthy immune system reaction resulting from injury to tissue. It is characterized by swelling and irritation of the surrounding area. It happens because capillaries that carry antibodies make themselves more permeable to let antibodies and repair cells get to the site of injury to get rid of pathogens and start the healing process. Discoverers of nanobacteria theorize that injuries caused by nanobacteria lead to a persistent inflammatory response, which is not healthy.

LDL – See Cholesterol.

Lipid – Medical term applied to some fats. Also includes some natural oils or waxes. Lipids are among the basic components in cells. They help give cells structure. They also store energy and carry vitamins.[7] Cholesterol and triglycerides are lipids. In heart disease lipids build up in the soft plaque that gums up blood vessels.

Macular Degeneration – A condition in which cells in a specific part of the eye degenerate, resulting in blurred vision and ultimately blindness. Calcification has been found in this disease.

MRI - Magnetic Resonance Imaging – A non-invasive procedure that uses powerful magnets and radio waves to construct pictures of the body. This is part of the growing group of technologies that show obstructions such as calcification and cancers. An MRA, or magnetic resonance angiogram, is a special type of magnetic resonance imaging which creates three-dimensional reconstructions of vessels containing flowing blood and is often utilized when conventional angiography cannot be performed.[8]

Mycoplasma – A sometimes toxic micro-organism that lacks a cell wall and that is so small it often gets through filters and contaminates the serum in which biological experiments are done. One species causes a type of pneumonia in humans.

Nano organism – There is no official definition for this, but here we use it to describe a life form that measures less than one millionth of a meter in diameter. Nanobacteria, for example, measure 50 – 250 nanometers in diameter.

Nanometer – One billionth of a meter.

PATCH study – PATCH stands for Program to Assess Alternative Treatment Strategies to Achieve Cardiac Health.[9] This name was applied to a controversial study done to evaluate the impacts of EDTA intravenous chelation on cardiovascular disease. Results of the study suggested no benefits arising from chelation, but the methodology has been criticized by chelation proponents. This controversy may be settled by a $30 million study being done by the National Institutes of Health.

Pathogen – An agent—usually a microorganism—that causes disease. Nanobacteria are considered to be pathogens.

Psoriasis – A noncontagious inflammatory skin disease characterized by recurring reddish patches covered with silvery scales. These scales contain calcium deposits.

Rapid CT Scan – See Electron Beam Computed Tomography.

Renal disease – Disease associated with the kidneys and often with calcification.

RNA (Ribonucleic acid) – Transmits genetic information in every cell. Essential for replication. RNA has been found in nanobacteria.

Scleroderma – A pathological thickening and hardening of the skin associated with calcification.

Sedimentation rate, or Erythrocyte sedimentation rate (ESR) – A non-specific screening test for various diseases. The test measures the distance that red blood cells settle in unclotted blood toward the bottom of a specially marked test tube in one hour. This is used to monitor inflammatory disease and is used as one measure of rheumatoid arthritis, heart, and kidney disease.[10]

Statins – A group of drugs used to lower bad cholesterol levels by inhibiting a key enzyme involved in the biosynthesis of cholesterol. Statins have also been discovered to slow the progression of calcification in arteries, but the key word here is "slow," rather than reverse. Statins have not been found to reverse the existing buildup of calcified deposits.[11]

Stent – A tube inserted into a blood vessel to restore blood flow when buildups block it. Unfortunately, stents often reblock. Some newer stents are being coated with antibiotics to prevent this. Results are being examined now. It has been theorized that nanobacteria cause stents to reblock.

Stress test – Also known as an Exercise Electrocardiogram, this test measures the heart's response to an increased demand for oxygen brought on by exercise. It is used as an indicator of cardiovascular disease.

Tetracycline – Broad spectrum antibiotic to fight bacterial infections. A yellow crystalline compound that is synthesized or derived from microorganisms known as Streptomyces. Researchers have found that tetracycline kills uncalcified nanobacteria and may also have other beneficial impacts on infection in heart disease.

Thrombosis – The obstruction of a blood vessel by a clot. Clotting is a healthy reaction of the body to injury, but it gets out of hand when it occurs in blocked blood vessels and often leads to death. Kajander and his colleagues found that nanobacteria seem to spark clotting in arteries because they bind a substance known as prothrombin.

Triglycerides – A type of fat produced by the body to store energy. It is measured as a mild risk factor for coronary artery disease. See also Lipid.

Ultra Fast or Rapid CT scan – See Electron Beam Computed Tomography.

Vascular disease – Blockage of blood vessels due to swelling, plaque, and hard deposits.

Vascular system – Network of vessels that carry blood or lymph through the body.

White blood cell count – A high white blood cell count indicates infection or inflammation that has activated the body's immune response. When taken with other test results, such as triglycerides and C-reactive protein, it can indicate inflammation in heart disease.

Who's Who In The World Of Calcification And Nanobacteria

Hundreds of researchers and physicians are now involved with nanobacteria and calcification. This list shows some of the major participants and their roles. It focuses on "blood nanobacteria" rather than the much larger world of nanobacteria outside the human body, although some players in the wider field are named.

Researchers

Arthur Agatston, M.D., F.A.C.C., Mt. Sinai Medical Center, Miami Beach, FL, USA: Developer of "the Agatston Score," a method for standardizing calcium scores on the ultra-fast scanning machines that are used to check for calcification.

Katja M. Aho, MSc., University of Kuopio, Department of Biochemistry, Kuopio, Finland: collaborates with Olavi Kajander on researching and describing the challenges associated with characterizing nanobacteria.

Kari K. Akerman, University of Kuopio, A. I. Virtanen Institute, Department of Biochemistry and Biotechnology, Kuopio, Finland: Collaborated with Olavi Kajander on Scanning Electron Microscopy in relation to nanobacteria.

Dennis A. Carson, M.D., Ph.D., University of California at San Diego, Former Dean, Faculty of Medicine. Director, the Sam and Rose Stein Institute for Research on Aging, La Jolla,

CA, USA: Member, National Academy of Sciences. Postulated that most extraskeletal calcification may be caused by nanobacteria.

David Y. Chan, M.D., Johns Hopkins Hospital, James Buchanan Brady Urological Institute, Baltimore, MD, USA: Urologist who did research on nanobacteria and formation of kidney stones.

Neva Çiftçioglu, Ph.D., Universities Space Research Association, Division of Space Life Sciences, Houston, TX, USA; Co-founded Nanobac Oy, Finland: Co-discoverer of methods for culturing and detecting nanobacteria. Plays a leading role in *Nanobacterium sanguineum* research. Made significant contributions by reducing the time it took to culture nanobacteria and by developing antibody methods to detect them in living mammals—such as humans.

Vefa Çiftçioglu, D.D.S., Ankara, Turkey: Co-published paper with his sister Neva Çiftçioglu on nanobacteria and dental stones.

Franklin Cockerill, Ph.D., M.D., Mayo Clinic, Chief of microbiology, infectious diseases, Rochester, MN, USA: Known for his work on anthrax vaccine. Heads a research team working on basic science of nanobacteria diagnostics and plans to sequence genome of nanobacteria.

Fredric Coe, M.D., Professor, University of Chicago, IL, USA: A leading urology researcher in elimination of kidney stones. Currently examining cause of calcification in kidney disease.

Paul W. Ewald, Ph.D., Amherst College, Amherst, NY, USA: Leading investigator into infection as a cause of heart and other diseases. Has published several books on the topic. Has spoken briefly on the potential role of nanobacteria in atherosclerosis.

Enrique Garcia-Cuerpo, M.D., Alcala University, Department of Medicine, Madrid, Spain: Co-published work on kidney stones and nanobacteria, especially relating to fulfillment of Koch's Postulates.

Rauno Harvima, M.D., Kuopio University Hospital, Department of Dermatology, Kuopio, Finland: Researches the relationship between dermatological calcification and nanobacteria in psoriasis, eczema, lichen planus, atopic dermatitis, and scleroderma.

J. Thomas Hjelle, Ph.D., University of Illinois College of Medicine at Peoria, Departments of Biomedical and Therapeutic Sciences, Peoria, IL, USA: Researches the role nanobacteria may play in Polycystic Kidney Disease and kidney stones, pineal calcification, and brain sand.

Martin Holmberg, M.D., Uppsala University, Department of Medical Sciences, Uppsala, Sweden: Swedish scientist working on nanobacteria detection in serum.

E. Olavi Kajander, M.D., Ph.D., Nanobac Oy, Kuopio, Finland; NanobacLabs Research Institute, Tampa, FL, USA: Discovered and patented *Nanobacterium sanguineum*. Along with his colleague Neva Çiftçioglu, he devised ways of culturing it and testing for it. Co-developed the NanobacTEST U/A with Dr. Gary Mezo. The leading basic science researcher in this field, and a practicing physician.

Ilpo Kuronen, University of Kuopio, A. I. Virtanen Institute, Department of Clinical Chemistry, Kuopio, Finland: Finnish co-researcher on nanobacteria.

Hilary M. Lapin-Scott, Ph.D., Professor, Exeter University, Biological Sciences, Exeter, United Kingdom: Lapin-Scott and her colleague S. Burton have researched culturability and biofilm formation related to nanobacteria.

John C. Lieske, M.D., Mayo Medical School, Assistant Professor of Medicine, Research Chair Division of Nephrology, Rochester, MN, USA: Works with multidisciplinary group at Mayo to study pathogenic role of nanobacteria in human disease, especially kidney stones, Polycystic Kidney Disease, and atherosclerosis.

Gary S. Mezo, A.R.N.P., P.A., N.D., Ph.D., Founder/ Chairman of Board, and Chief Research Officer, Nanobac Pharmaceuticals Inc. and NanobacLabs Research Institute, Tampa, FL, USA. The top nanobacteria treatment developer. Invented and developed the prescription nanobiotic NanobacTX, the first treatment deliberately targeted at eliminating nanobacteria in the human body. Co-developed the NanobacTEST U/A with Dr. Kajander. Initiated the first independently verified clinical studies on the medical impacts of NanobacTX, UroBac and DermaBac, and other nanobiotics. His NanobacLabs Research Institute is the leading research organization for nanobiotic therapies and diagnostics. He has acquired Nanobac Oy, a leading nanobacteria testing laboratory based in Finland.

Alan Miller, M.D., Professor of Medicine, University of Florida Health Science Center, Division of Cardiology, Jacksonville, FL, USA: Served on cardiology review board for the first clinical study of the effects of the nanobiotic NanobacTX in heart patients (NanobacTX-ACESII Cardiology Study).

Virginia M. Miller, Ph.D., Professor of Surgery, Professor of Physiology, Mayo Medical School, Rochester, MN, USA: Researches the relationship between arteriosclerosis and nanobacteria. Co-published studies on detection of nanobacteria in arteriosclerotic plaque.

Marcia Miller-Hjelle, Ph.D., A.B.M.M., University of Illinois College of Medicine at Peoria, Departments of Biomedical and Therapeutic Sciences, Peoria, IL, USA: Researches the role nanobacteria may play in Polycystic Kidney Disease and kidney stones, pineal calcification and brain sand.

László Puskás, Ph.D., Hungarian Academy of Science, DNA-Chip Laboratory, Biological Research Center, Szeged, Hungary: First isolated nanobacteria from arteriosclerotic plaque.

Todd E. Rasmussen, M.D., Mayo Clinic and Foundation, Rochester, MN, USA: Co-researches nanobacteria in arteriosclerotic plaque with Austin Heart Center at the University of Texas.

George P. Rodgers, M.D., F.A.C.C., University of Texas, Austin Heart Center, Austin, TX, USA: Co-researches nanobacteria in arteriosclerotic plaque with Mayo Clinic.

Vardit Segal, Technion-Israel Institute of Technology, Leonard & Diane Sherman Center for Research in Biomaterials, Department of Biomedical Engineering, Haifa, Israel: Co-published with Dr. Kajander about nanobacteria forming apatite coating.

Andrei P. Sommer, Ph.D., University of Ulm, Central Institute of Biomedical Engineering, Ulm, Germany: Co-published with Kajander about nanobacteria and kidney stone formation, and light-induced replication of nanobacteria. Expert in Near-Field Optical Analysis.

Eduardo Turcott, McGill University, Electron Microscopy Centre, Montreal, Canada: Co-researches nanobacteria in dental pulp.

Hojatollah Vali, Ph.D., Director, McGill University, Electron Microscopy Centre, Montreal, Canada: Researches nanobacteria and worked with McKay and Çiftçioglu's team on the Martian meteorite. Co-published on nanobacteria in dental pulp.

Testing labs

Many clinical labs are being used throughout the world to test for nanobacteria, but **Nanobac OY,** based in Finland, is the pioneering one. It was first to develop tests for detecting nanobacteria. Its methods form the basis for methods that commercial labs use for detecting nanobacteria infections. It was started by Drs. Olavi Kajander and Neva Çiftçioglu and is controlled by Nanobac Pharmaceuticals Inc., Tampa, Florida.

Nanobacteria critics

Charles F.A. Bryce, Professor, Braids Education Consultants, Edinburgh, Scotland: Published a paper claiming that apatite crystals have been mistaken for nanobacteria.

John O. Cisar, Ph.D., National Institutes of Health, National Institute of Dental and Craniofacial Research, Oral Infection and Immunity Branch, Bethesda, MD, USA: Published research questioning the existence of nanobacteria as free living organisms.

Elmer M. Cranton, M.D., family practice physician, Mount Rainier Clinic, Yelm, WA, USA: IV Chelation expert who challenges evidence that nanobacteria cause arteriosclerotic plaque.

Jouni Issakainen, Mycologist, Turku University Central Hospital, Turku, Finland: Sparked public scientific fraud investigation against Dr. Kajander in Finland [Kajander was later unconditionally cleared when the investigating committee dismissed the claims as groundless].

Dennis J. Kopecko, Ph.D., Chief, Laboratory of Enteric and Sexually Transmitted Diseases, Food and Drug Administration, Rockville, MD, USA: Collaborated with Cisar on nanobacteria research. Says they found no credible molecular evidence to support the existence of nanobacteria.

Related research on other types of nano-organisms such as nan[n]obacteria / archaeae / nanobes

Robert L. Folk, Ph.D., Professor Emeritus, University of Texas, Department of Geological Sciences, Austin, TX, USA: Folk is one of the first to describe nano-scale bacteria-like organisms in geological specimens. Years later he participated in a study by the Mayo Clinic and University of Texas in 2002 that confirmed the original work by Dr. László Puskás on existence of nanobacteria in arterial plaque that characterizes heart disease.

Brenda L. Kirkland, Ph.D., Mississippi State University, Strakville, MS, USA: Geologist who works with and co-published with Robert Folk.

David McKay, Ph.D., NASA Lyndon B. Johnson Space Center, Space and Life Science Directorate, Houston, TX, USA: Director of a section of the Mars Program at NASA that focuses on potential life forms on Mars. Published controversial paper showing evidence of life in Martian meteorite. He brought the work of Neva Çiftçioglu to the attention of NASA, after which she was invited by the agency to help them investigate nanobacteria. McKay has been a staunch defender of Kajander's and Çiftçioglu's work.

Richard Y. Morita: First used the term "nannobacteria" with two N's in a 1988 paper.[1] He has also written a book on nutrient-poor environments in which nanobacteria may thrive.[2]

Karl Stetter, Ph.D., Professor, University of Regensburg, Regensburg, Germany: Discoverer of nanoscale bacteria-like organisms in volcanic vents in Iceland in 2001 that may be related to the geological entities discovered ten years earlier by Robert Folk. Has done groundbreaking work on DNA analysis of the organisms.

Philippa Uwins, Ph.D., Senior Research Fellow, University of Queensland, Centre for Microscopy and Microanalysis, St. Lucia, Australia: Uwins and colleagues A. Taylor and R. Webb have published about their research on "nanobes" and into lower size limits of life. Dr. Uwins' team has resisted calling her discovery "nanobacteria." Instead they have given them the name of "nanobes" until more is discovered and researched.

Journalists who have covered nanobacteria

Alison Abbott, Ph.D., Senior European correspondent *Nature* Magazine, Munich, Germany: Covers controversial stories in the field of genetics. She wrote stories in 1999 and 2000 about the academic fraud accusation against Dr. Kajander, but she has not yet updated the story about his having been cleared of the charges.

W. Allan Hamilton, Ph.D., Professor, University of Aberdeen, Institute of Medical Sciences, Department of Molecular & Cell Biology, Aberdeen, United Kingdom: Produced a summary article on the debates summarizing whether nanobacteria are alive or not.

Stephen Hart: Has written numerous informative articles on nanobacteria in Astrobiology magazine.

Douglas Mulhall: Has written articles about *Nanobacterium sanguineum*, and was the first to discuss the nanobiotic treatment for nanobacteria in his book, *Our Molecular Future: How Nanotechnology, Robotics, Genetics, and Artificial Intelligence Will Transform Our World* (Amherst, NY: Prometheus Books, 2002)

Sonya Pemberton, Karena Slaninka, Filmmakers: Wrote, directed and produced "Alien Underworld" (Tattooed Media, 2002), one of the first televised documentaries about nanobacteria. First broadcast in Australia.

Cynthia Smoot, FOX TV reporter in Tampa, FL, USA: Produced documentary on nanobiotics featuring Drs. Mezo, Kajander, and Maniscalco.

Michael Ray Taylor: Published what is arguably the first book about nanobacteria: *Dark Life – Martian Nanobacteria, Rock Eating Cave Bugs and Other Extreme Organisms of Inner Earth and Outer Space* (New York: Scribner, 1999).

Insurance

Alan Iezzi, M.D., F.A.A.F.P., Founder, Patient-Directed Care, Tampa, FL, USA: Medical director of a healthcare company that is embarking on a program to let patients select their own treatments based on a discount system that removes insurers from making decisions for patients and doctors. Plans to include nanobiotics in the program.

Some Practicing Physicians

Robert C. Atkins, M.D., F.A.C.C., Cardiologist, Founder of the Atkins Center for Cardiology: Author of many books. Participated in the NanobacTX ACES Multicenter Study. He died accidentally in 2003.

Patrick Fratellone, M.D., F.A.C.C., Executive Medical Director of The Fratellone Group for Integrative Cardiology and Medicine, New York, NY, USA: Medical practice focuses on two epidemics: Diabetes and Obesity. Participated in the first NanobacTX ACES Multicenter Study. Currently participating in Nanobac Pharmaceuticals study of nanobiotic treatment in cardiac patients with diabetes.

Benedict S. Maniscalco, M.D., F.A.C.C., Tampa, FL, USA: One of America's leading cardiologists who supervised the first formal clinical study of heart patients taking nanobiotics, the NanobacTX-ACES II.

James C. Roberts Jr., M.D., F.A.C.C., Comprehensive Heart Care - EECP Center of Northwest Ohio, Toledo, USA: An experienced practitioner of EECP therapy as described in this book. One of the first of many cardiologists to prescribe

NanobacTX. Has developed considerable experience with the nanobiotic therapy. His website (www.heartfixer.com) contains among the most comprehensive independent analysis' available. Participated in the NanobacTX-ACES Multicenter Study.

Daniel A. Shoskes, M.D., F.R.C.S., Director of Renal Transplant, Cleveland Clinic Florida, Department of Urology, Weston, FL, USA: Has written leading papers on the role of biofilm and calcification in prostatitis. He is also investigating potential impacts of nanobiotics on disease in patients.

Stephen Sinatra, M.D., F.A.C.C., F.A.C.N., New England Heart and Longevity Center, Manchester, CT, USA: One of the pioneering physicians who prescribed NanobacTX.

Daniel N. Tucker, M.D., Allergist & Immunologist, West Palm Beach, FL, USA: Prescribing physician who is optimistic about the nanobiotic treatment but reserves judgement on what exactly nanobacteria may prove to be.

How Nanobacteria May Trigger The Atherosclerotic Process

This "plain language" outline of the role of nanobacteria in atherosclerosis was written in consultation with Drs. Gary Mezo, Neva Çiftçioglu, Olavi Kajander, and Benedict Maniscalco. It is still a "work in progress" that may constitute the beginnings of a unifying theory of how coronary and other types of heart disease develop.

There are many possible pathways for nanobacteria to enter the human body. Here is a sequence where nanobacteria enter the body via contaminated vaccines, blood transfusion, contaminated water, or other possible sources. The process described below may take years or decades:

1. Nanobacteria enter the bloodstream directly, or pass through the digestive system. They are carried throughout the capillaries, veins, and arteries. They replicate once every 3-6 days and grow by using calcium, phosphate, and lipids available in the blood.

2. At this stage the body can still get rid of many nanobacteria. They are excreted harmlessly into the urine. However, a few may get stuck in the kidney filtration system walls. Others are carried in the blood and get stuck in arteries and veins where flow is reduced at a splitting, bend, or narrowing in capillary beds of tissue, or at a site of injury or tumor growth.

3. As they grow, nanobacteria form colonies and secrete biofilm. The slimy biofilm helps nanobacteria work together as a group and get food. It also helps the colonies to invade healthy cells. Later, it will help to build a hard protective shell. The multiple roles of this biofilm as a smokescreen, toxin, and defense are specific to nanobacteria.

4. Nanobacteria cause death to cells that internalize them. It is believed by the researchers that the human body has only a limited capacity to kill them. It tries to wall them off but this only slows their growth when they are in calcified form, and may also exacerbate the process of calcification. As the colony grows, signs of persistent infection arise and the body's defenses go into more aggressive action. White blood cells begin to attack the colony. They are triggered by the presence of toxins generated by nanobacteria and by inflammatory signals from cells. This is accelerated by premature death of cells from invasion of the nanobacteria.

    In response to the white blood cell attacks, nanobacteria shield themselves by secreting more slimy biofilm. Fatty streaks form on this battlefield as a byproduct of the "inflammatory cascade" response. This is an extraordinarily complex process.

5. The body surrounds the area of nanobacterial infection much in the same way that it does a cyst. The available nutrient supply for the nanobacteria begins to diminish. This is where a special property of nanobacteria comes into play. The colonies secrete calcium phosphate to build a sticky slime that hardens into an igloo-like shell that encases them. One shell can grow to be about 2-3 microns in diameter and may contain several specialized "mother" units. These may later spin off thousands of smaller nanobacteria known as "buds". Millions of shells aggregate to form calcified deposits that over time will be visible and quantifiable on a rapid CT scan.

6. The encased nanobacteria go into semi-hibernation, but continue to grow their shells and also produce buds of tiny nanobacteria. Thus, the calcium deposit continues to grow upon itself "coral-like". This process occurs more slowly than replication of un-encased nanobacteria, but it still continues relentlessly.

7. At this point, nanobacteria can be found in different stages throughout the body: Growing, replicating, secreting biofilm, semi-hibernating in shells, and producing buds while being calcified and walled off within arteries and veins.

8. Meanwhile, the wall of the artery where the nanobacteria colony is located has been swelling in an inflammatory response to this infection. An inflammatory response occurs when tissues are injured by bacteria, toxins, or another cause. Damaged tissue releases chemicals that cause blood vessels to leak fluid and stimulate localized swelling. This helps to isolate the foreign substance from further contact with body tissues. The inflammatory response also attracts an invasion of "host cells" to the area. Together, these processes initiate the formation of a complex group of fatty, fibrous, and calcified deposits, otherwise referred to as "plaque." The calcified deposits in atherosclerotic plaques form about twenty per cent of this mass.

9. After many years, the growing plaque reduces the diameter of blood vessels. As our immune system continues to try and clean up the infection, the composition of the plaque changes. The relative amount of soft plaque decreases while "hard" plaque generated by nanobacterial calcification increases. At the same time, the body tries to bore new blood vessels into the plaque. Inadvertently, this feeds more nutrients to the semi-dormant nanobacteria, reviving them and causing their activity to accelerate, resulting in new inflammatory responses.

10. The process of nanobacteria replication repeats itself in many more locations. Deposits may form in the

kidneys to trigger kidney stones, or the eyes to build cataracts. They may lodge in the muscles or joints to initiate arthritis-like or fibromyalgia-like symptoms.

11.   This massive invasion triggers a chronic inflammatory response throughout the body, sending the immune system into a life-long overdrive that ultimately will cause a crisis.

12.   Eventually an artery clogs, or the artery wall ruptures as it becomes brittle, then stretches, causing a clot that leads to death or heart failure. Clotting is a problem because nanobacteria seem to bind together with prothrombin, the chemical that generates clots.

13.   If a surgical procedure such as angioplasty is used on blood vessels, it releases billions of nanobacteria when their shelters are "smashed" and the nanobacteria are exposed to nutrient-rich blood again. This kick-starts their cycle, causing an acute "inflammatory cascade." They begin to replicate rapidly. The body's defenses cannot cope, and a crisis may occur.

Bibliography

Aside from papers shown here, others are referenced in the endnotes that in some cases show websites where the papers can be located.

Academic Research Papers

Ackerman, K., and I. Kuronen, E.O. Kajander. "Scanning Electron Microscopy of Nanobacteria-Novel Biofilm Producing Organisms in Blood." *Scanning* 15, III (1993).

Breitschwerdt, E., and S. Sontakke, A. Cannedy, S. Hancock, J. Bradley. "Infection with *Bartonella weissii* and Detection of *Nanobacterium sanguineum* Antigens in a North Carolina Beef Herd." *Journal of Clinical Microbiology* 39, no. 3 (Mar. 2001): 879-82.

Bryce, Charles F. A. "Alternative View on the Putative Organism, *Nanobacterium sanguineum*," Braids Education Consultants, Edinburgh EH10 6NZ, Scotland (Undated) [online], http://www.heartfixer.com/Nanobacterium-Report.htm [January 23, 2003].

Carr, S., and A. Farb, W. Pearce, *et al.* "Activated Inflammatory Cells are Associated with Plaque Rupture in Carotid Artery Stenosis." *Surgery* 122 (1997): 757-63.

Çiftçioglu, N., and E. O. Kajander. "Interaction of Nanobacteria with Cultured Mammalian Cells." *Pathophysiology* 4 (1998): 259-70.

Çiftçioglu, N., and M. A. Miller-Hjelle, J. T. Hjelle, E. O. Kajander. "Inhibition of Nanobacteria by Antimicrobial Drugs as Measured by a Modified Microdilution Method." *Antimicrobial Agents and Chemotherapy* 46 (July 2002): 2077-86.

Çiftçioglu, Neva, and David S. McKay, E. Olavi Kajander. "Association Between Nanobacteria and Periodontal Disease," *Circulation* 108 (August 2003): 58-9.

Cisar, John O., and De-Qi Xu, John Thompson, William Swaim, Lan Hu, Dennis J. Kopecko. "An Alternative Interpretation of Nanobacteria-induced Biomineralization." *Proceedings of the National Academy of Sciences* 97 (10 October 2000): 11511-15.

Freimuth, V., and H. Linnan, P. Polyxeni. "Communicating the Threat of Emerging Infections to the Public." *CDC Emerging Infectious Diseases* 6, no. 4 (2000).

Garcia-Cuerpo, E., and E. O. Kajander, N. Çiftçioglu, F. Lovaco-Castellano *et al.* "Nanobacteria: An Experimental Neo-Lithogenesis Model." *Arch Esp Urol.* 53, no. 4 (May 2000): 291-303.

Greenwald, R. "Treatment of Destructive Arthritic Disorders with MMP Inhibitors." *Ann NY Acad Sci* 732 (1994): 199-205.

Hjelle, T., and M. Miller-Hjelle, I. Poxton, E. O. Kajander, N. Çiftçioglu, *et al.* "Endotoxin & Nanobacteria in Polycystic Kidney Disease." International Society of Nephrology; *Kidney International* 57 (2000): 2360-74.

Holvoet, P., *et al.* "Circulating Oxidized LDL a Sensitive Marker of CAD." *Arterioscler Thromb Vasc Biol* 21 (2001): 844-48.

Houpikian, Pierre and Didier Raoult. "Traditional and Molecular Techniques for the Study of Emerging Bacterial Diseases: One Laboratory's Perspective." *Emerging Infectious Diseases* 8, no. 2 (February 2002).

Jantos, C., and A. Nesseler, W. Waas, *et al.* "Low Prevalence of *Chlamydia pneumoniae* in Atherectomy Specimens from Patients with Coronary Heart Disease." *Clin Infect Dis* 28, no. 5 (1999): 988-92.

Joseph, A., D. Ackerman, J. Talley, *et al.* "Manifestations of Coronary Atherosclerosis in Young Trauma Victims:

An Autopsy Study." *J Am Coll Cardiol* 22 (1993): 459-67.

Kajander, E. O., and K. Aho, V. Segal. "Apatite Biofilm Forming Agent: Nanobacteria as a Model System for Biomineralization and Biological Standard for NOA. A Preliminary Study." Proceedings of the 2nd International Conference on Near-Field Optical Analysis: Photodynamic Therapy & Photobiology Effects, Houston, TX (30.05. – 01.06.01). NASA/CP 210786 (October 2002): 51-57.

Kajander, E. O., and N. Çiftçioglu, K. Aho, E. Carcia-Cuerpo. "Characteristics of Nanobacteria and Their Possible Role in Stone Formation." Invited Editorial. *Urological Research* 31, 2 (Jun. 2003): 47-54.

Kajander, E. O., and N. Çiftçioglu, M. Miller-Hjelle, T. Hjelle, "Nanobacteria: Controversial Pathogens in Nephrolithiasis and Polycystic Kidney Disease." *Current Opinion Nephrology and Hypertension* 10 (May 2001): 445-52.

Kweider, M., and G. Lowe, G. Murray, D. Kinane, D. McGowan. "Dental Disease, Fibrinogen and White Cell Count: Links with Myocardial Infarction." *Scottish Med J* 38, no. 3 (Jun. 1993): 73-74.

Li, Y., and Y. Wen, Z. Yang, H. Wei, W. Liu, A. Tan, X. Wu, Q. Wang, S. Huang, E. O. Kajander, N. Çiftçioglu. "Culture and Identification of Nanobacteria in Bile." *Zhonghua Yi Xue Za Zhi* 25 (2002): 1557-60. Article in Chinese. In this work 61% of 75 patient bile samples removed during cholecystectomy were positive for nanobacteria with culture and TEM and with a novel calcification assay.

Libby, P., and D. Egan, S. Skarlatos. "Roles of Infectious Agents in Atherosclerosis and Restenosis." *Circulation* 96 (1997): 4095-103.

Lopez-Brea, M., and R. Selgas. "Nanobacteria as a Cause of Renal Diseases and Vascular Calcifying Pathology in Renal Patients ("Endovascular Lithiasis")." *Enferm Infec Microbiol Clin* 18, no. 10 (Dec. 2000): 491-92.

Miller-Hjelle, M. A., and J. T. Hjelle, N. Çiftçioglu and E. O. Kajander. "Nanobacteria. Methods for Growth and Identification of this Recently Discovered Calciferous Agent. In: *Rapid Microbiological Methods for the 21th Cen-*

tury. Ed. W. Olson. Raleigh N.C.: Davis Horwood Int. Publishers, in press March 2003.

Nazir, R., and S. Gupta. "Clinical Significance of Coronary Calcification." *Emer Med* (Feb. 2001): 107-10.

O'Rourke, R. A., *et al.* "American College of Cardiology/American Heart Association Expert Consensus Document on Electronbeam Computed Tomography for Diagnosis and Prognosis of Coronary Artery Disease." *J Am Coll Cardiol* 36 (2000): 326.

Pasterkamp, G., and A. Schoneveld, A. C. van del Wal, *et al.* "Inflammation of the Atherosclerotic Cap and Shoulder of the Plaque is a Common and Locally Observed Feature in Unruptured Plaques of Femoral and Coronary Arteries." *Arterioscler Thromb Vasc Biol* 19 (1999): 54-58.

Ray, J., and W. Stetler-Stevenson. "The Role of Matrix Metalloproteinases and Their Inhibitors in Tumor Invasion, Metastasis and Angiogenesis." *Eur Res J* 7 (1994): 2062-72.

Rifai, N., and R. Joubran, H. Yu, *et al.* "Inflammatory Markers in Men with Angiographically Documented Coronary Heart Disease." *Clin Chem* 45 (1999): 1967-73.

Rumberger, J., and D. Simons, L. Fitzpatrick, *et al.* "Coronary Artery Calcium Area by Electron Beam Computed Tomography and Coronary Atherosclerotic Plaque Area: a Histopathologic Correlative Study." *Circulation* 92 (1995): 2157-62.

Sangiorgi, G., and J. Rumberger, A. Severson, *et al.* "Arterial Calcification and NOT Lumen Stenosis is Highly Correlated with Atherosclerotic Plaque Burdens in Humans: a Histologic Study of 723 Coronary Artery Segments Using Nondecalcifying Methodology." *J Am Coll Cardiol* 31 (1998): 126-33.

Sommer, A. P., and H. Hassinen, E. O. Kajander. "Light Induced Replication of Nanobacteria – A preliminary Report." *J. Clin. Laser Med. Surg.* 20 (2002): 241-44.

Sommer, A. P., and E. O. Kajander. "Nanobacteria-induced Kidney Stone Formation: Novel Paradigm Based on the FERMIC Model." *Crystal Growth & Design* 2 (2002): 563-65.

Sommer, A. P., and David S. McKay, Neva Çiftçioglu, Uri Oron, Adam R. Mester, E. Olavi Kajander. "Living Nanovesicles: Chemical and Physical Survival Strategies of Primordial Biosystems. Living Nanovesicles Perspectives." *Journal of Proteome Research* 2, no.4 (Jul.-Aug. 2003): 441-43.

Sommer, A. P., and U. Oron, E. O. Kajander, A. R. Mester. "Stressed Cells Survive Better With Light." *Journal of Proteome Research* 1 (2002): 475.

Vainshtein, M., and E. Kudriashova. "Nanobacteria." *Mikrobiologiia* 69, no. 2 (2000): 163-74.

van der Wal, A. C., and A. Becker, C. M. van der Loos, *et al.* "Site of Intimal Rupture or Erosion of Thrombosed Coronary Atherosclerotic Plaques is Characterized by an Inflammatory Process Irrespective of the Dominant Plaque Morphology." *Circulation* 89 (1994): 36-44.

Books

Most of the information for this book was gleaned from scientific publications, subject interviews, and correspondence rather than books, because while thousands of books deal with heart disease or diets to prevent it, relatively few deal with calcification. Some books that deal with pathological calcification are out of print. The authors scanned dozens of diet books for mentions of "calcification," but we do not list most of them here since they do not contain relevant information about pathological calcification, its cause, or possible remedy. Therefore the book list in this section is short.

Atkins, Robert C. *Dr. Atkins' New Diet Revolution.* New York: Avon Books, 1999 (revised 2003).

Dvonch, Louis A., and Russell Dvonch. *The Heart Attack Germ.* New York: Writer's Showcase, 2003.

Ewald, Paul W. *Evolution of Infectious Diseases.* New York: Oxford University Press, 1994.

Ewald, Paul W. *Plague Time, The New Germ Theory of Disease.* London: Anchor Books, 2002.

Garrett, Laurie. *Betrayal of Trust, The Collapse of Global Public Health.* New York: Hyperion, 2001.

Mulhall, Douglas. *Our Molecular Future: How Nanotechnology, Robotics, Genetics, and Artificial Intelligence Will Transform Our World.* Amherst NY: Prometheus, 2002.

Null, Gary. *Seven Steps to Perfect Health.* Austin TX: I Books, 2001.

Ornish, Dean. *Dr. Dean Ornish's Program for Reversing Heart Disease.* New York: Ballantine, 1992 (revised 2003).

Taylor, Michael Ray. *Dark Life: Martian Nanobacteria, Rock-eating Cave Bugs, and Other Extreme Organisms of Inner Earth and Outer Space.* New York: Scribner, 1999.

Helpful Websites

There are dozens of websites about calcification, nanobacteria, nanobes, and "nannobacteria," and thousands of websites on the diseases related to them. Here are a few directory websites that lead to many of them. Please refer to the websites shown in the endnotes for information about calcification-related illnesses.

http://www.calcify.com – Homepage for this book. Provides updates to information from the book, supplementary data, links to other websites, and reviews of the book. The site changes often as information becomes available.

http://www.NanobacLabs.com – Homepage of Nanobac Pharmaceuticals Inc. in Tampa, Florida, the company that invented nanobiotics, developed NanobacTX and other prescription drugs, and offers the only valid test kits for detecting nanobacteria. Contains up-to-date information on studies and treatments. Very good for background information on the researchers as well. Also the homepage for the NanobacLabs Research Institute.

http://www.heartfixer.com/indexNB.htm – Nanobacteria section of the website of Ohio-based Dr. James C. Roberts, one of the first cardiologists to prescribe NanobacTX. Valuable case studies.

http://www.nanobac.com – Homepage of Nanobac Oy, a European subsidiary of Nanobac Pharmaceuticals Inc. Based in Kuopio, Finland. Developed the tests for nanobacteria.

http://www.noaw.com/Nanobacteria/nanobacteria.htm – Nanobacteria section of Network for Effective Women's Services (NEWS) based in Watkinsville, Georgia. Has good summary of links to nanobacteria web sites.

http://www.thenanotechnologygroup.org/id71.htm – Webpage with a case history as told by a cataract patient.

http://www.lifescore.com – Homepage of a San Diego based clinic offering treatment for nanobacteria infections.

http://www.uq.edu.au/nanoworld/uwins.html – Webpage of Dr. Philippa Uwins at University of Queensland in Australia that describes the geological forms that she has named "nanobes." Good links to other stories.

http://www.astrobio.net – Astrobiology magazine, does occasional articles on nanobacteria.

Notes

Introduction

1. The form of cardiovascular disease referred to in most of this book is "hardening of the arteries," which is the popular term applied to *arteriosclerosis* and *atherosclerosis*. These two names are often used interchangeably and can therefore be confusing. "Athero"-sclerosis is a disease in which complex calcium and fatty material are deposited on the wall of the arteries. This narrows the arteries and eventually restricts blood flow. It is one of several types of "Arterio"-sclerosis, a disease characterized by thickening and hardening of artery walls. Conditions associated with the disease include: Aneurism, calcified heart valves, congestive heart failure, enlargement of the heart, known as cardiomegaly, heart attack, high blood pressure, stroke, and thrombosis (blood clots).

2. "Coronary Artery Disease," *The Harvard Medical School Family Health Guide*, New York Simon & Schuster, 1999, updated 2003 [online], http://www.health.harvard.edu/fhg/fhgupdate/K/K2.shtml [April 14, 2003].

3. "Of more than 50 million deaths worldwide in 1997, about one-third were due to infectious and parasitic diseases such as acute lower respiratory diseases, tuberculosis, diarrhea, HIV/AIDS and malaria; about 30% were due to circulatory diseases such as coronary heart disease and cerebrovascular diseases (auth. note: both are caused by atherosclerosis), and about 12% were due to cancers. While deaths due to circulatory diseases declined from 51% to 46% of total deaths in the developed world during the period 1985-1997, they increased from 16% to 24% of total deaths in the developing world." *The World Health Report 1998*: *Ex-*

ecutive Summary, World Health Organization [online], http://www.who.int/whr2001/2001/archives/1998/exsum98e.htm [January 27, 2003].

4. Alexander Fleming is credited with discovering penicillin in 1928, but only after many approaches had been tried by other researchers. Some methods such as sterilization had shown earlier but limited success. It took other scientists such as Howard Florey to find ways of mass manufacturing the drug many years later before it could come into broad use in World War II.

5. As we'll see later in this book, this "newly isolated" pathogen was discovered in 1985, but was not isolated in heart disease until the late 1990's. News of such isolation was only published in 2002.

Chapter 1   When To Say "I'm Cured"

1. It was theorized as early as 1500 by Italian physician Girolamo Fracastoro that invisible organisms cause disease, but it wasn't until the 1850s that researchers such as Ignaz Semelweis, John Snow, and Heinrich Anton deBary began to demonstrate the link between bacteria and disease. Lansing M. Prescott, Donald A. Klein, John P. Harley, *Microbiology*. McGraw Hill Learning Center 2002 [online], http://highered.mcgraw-hill.com/sites/0072320419/student_view0/interactive_time_line.html [April 2, 2003].

2. Ibid. In 1867 Joseph Lister published the first work on antiseptic surgery, launching the trend toward aseptic techniques in medicine.

3. In 1815 "London surgeon Joseph Hodgson published an important monograph on vascular disease, claiming that inflammation was the underlying cause of atherosclerosis and it is not a natural degenerative occurrence of the aging process." Mohammad Madjid, "Milestones in Atherosclerosis and Vulnerable Plaque," Association for the Eradication of Heart Attack, 2002 [online], http://www.vp.org/Milestones/Milestones.htm [March 29, 2003]. Then in 1976 Russell Ross theorized that heart disease was an inflammatory response to injury from disease. This work was updated in: R. Ross, "Mechanisms of Disease: Atherosclerosis – An Inflammatory Disease," [Review Article], *New England Journal of Medicine* 340 (1999): 115-26.

4. See Introduction note 1, and the Glossary for descriptions of heart disease and arteriosclerosis.

5. A check of many medical dictionaries, cancer websites, and infectious disease books will show variations on the technical definition of being "cured."

6. "A Cure For Cardiovascular Disease?" Editorial, *British Medical Journal* 326 (June 28, 2003):1407-08.

7. Emma Ross, "Combination Pill Could Cut Heart Attacks And Strokes By About 80 Percent, Scientists Say," *The Associated Press*, June 26, 2003,

8. David Satcher, "America Takes Heart Disease To Heart," Surgeon General, U.S. Department Of Health And Human Services, January 24-28 2000 [online], http://www.health.gov/Partnerships/Media/heart.htm [January 27, 2003].

9. Ron Winslow, "New Stents A Boon For Patients May Affect Rising Health Costs," *Wall Street Journal*, December 24, 2002, p.1.

10. See Glossary.

11. Robert C. Atkins, *Dr. Atkins' New Diet Revolution* (New York: Avon Books, 1999) (revised 2003). Arthur Agatston, *The South Beach Diet: The Delicious, Doctor-Designed, Foolproof Plan for Fast and Healthy Weight Loss* (New York: Rodale Press, 2003). These diets are each popular and have some similarities, but they differ in their approaches to, for example, carbohydrates.

12. Dean Ornish, *Dr. Dean Ornish's Program for Reversing Heart Disease* (New York: Ballantine, 1992) (revised 2003). Ornish has criticized the Atkins Diet approach.

13. "Questions & Answers: The NIH Trial of EDTA Chelation Therapy for Coronary Artery Disease," National Center for Complementary Medicine (August 7, 2002) [online], http://nccam.nih.gov/news/2002/chelation/q-and-a.htm [March 30, 2003].

14. Nobel laureate Linus Pauling's theory of heart disease claims that high doses of substances called Lp(a) binding inhibitors prevent and dissolve the atherosclerotic plaques of heart disease. M. Rath, L. Pauling, "Solution of the Puzzle of Human Cardiovascular Disease: Its primary cause is ascorbate deficiency, leading to the deposition of lipoprotein(a) and fibrinogen/fibrin in the vascular wall," *Journal of Orthomolecular Med* 6 (1991):125-34.

15. Louis A. Dvonch and Russell Dvonch, *The Heart Attack Germ* (Lincoln, NE: I-universe, 2003).

16. A. Raza-Ahmad, G.A. Klassen, D.A. Murphy, J.A. Sullivan, C.E. Kinley, R.W. Landymore, J.R. Wood, "Evidence of Type 2 Herpes Simplex Infection in Human Coronary Arteries at the Time of Coronary Artery Bypass Surgery," *Canadian Journal of Cardiology* 11, no. 11 (December 1995): 1025-29 [online], http://www.pulsus.com/CARDIOL/11_11/Raza_ed.htm [April 3, 2003].

17. This table draws from information provided in: K. Bachmaier, J. Le, J.M. Penninger, "Catching Heart Disease: Antigenic Mimicry and Bacterial Infections," *Nature Medicine* 6 (2000): 841-42. See also: Aristo Vojdani, "A Look at Infectious Agents as a Possible Causative Factor in Cardiovascular Disease," *Laboratory Medicine* 34, no. 4&5 (April/May 2003).

18. One example: Louis A. Dvonch and Russell Dvonch, *The Heart Attack Germ* (Lincoln, NE: I-universe, 2003). This book rightly identifies the signs of infection that have been emerging in heart disease, then claims that there is proof to show the role of *Chlamydia pneumonia* and other germs as the cause.

19. Christopher M. O'Connor, Michael W. Dunne, Marc A. Pfeffer, Joseph B. Muhlestein, Louis Yao, Sandeep Gupta, Rebecca J. Benner, Marian R. Fisher, Thomas D. Cook, "Azithromycin for the Secondary Prevention of Coronary Heart Disease Events," *Journal of the American Medical Association (JAMA)* 290, no. 11 (Sep. 2003): 1459-66.

20. "Inflammation, Heart Disease and Stroke: The Role of C-Reactive Protein," American Heart Association [online], http://www.americanheart.org/presenter.jhtml?identifier=4648 [April 3, 2003].

21. Ibid.

22. "Helicobacter pylori in Peptic Ulcer Disease," *NIH Consensus Statement Online 1994* (February 7-9, 1994) 12(1): 1-23 [online], http://consensus.nih.gov/cons/094/094_statement.htm [January 23, 2003].

23. "Population studies have indicated a 1.5 to 2.0-times greater risk of fatal cardiovascular disease in patients with periodontal disease. In study after study, a positive connection has been found between oral disease and cardiovascular health." From "Oral Disease and Systemic Health: What is the Connection?" American Association of Endodontists [online], http://www.aae.org/ss00ecfe.html [April 4, 2003].

24. Paul Khairy, Stephane Rinfret, Jean-Claude Tardif, Richard Marchand, Stan Shapiro, James Brophy, Jocelyn Dupuis, "Absence of Association Between Infectious Agents and Endothelial Function in Healthy Young Men," *Circulation* 107 (2003): 1966-71.

25. C. Espinola-Klein, H. J. Rupprecht, S. Blankenberg, C. Bickel, H. Kopp, A. Victor, G. Hafner, W. Prellwitz, W. Schlumberger, J. Meyer, "Impact of Infectious Burden on Progression of Carotid Atherosclerosis," *Stroke* 33, no. 11 (Nov. 2002): 2581-86.

26. Harvey McConnel, "Current Antibiotic Trials Test Role of Bacteria in Atherosclerosis," Doctor's Guide, August 1, 2002 [online] http://www.docguide.com/news/content.nsf/news/

8525697700573E1885256b51006ce88f?OpenDocument&id=
48DDE4A73E09A9698526880078C249&c=Bacterial
%20Infections&count=10 [April 17, 2003] reviewing Maija
Leinonen, Pekka Saikku, "Evidence for Infectious Agents in Cardiovascular Disease and Atherosclerosis," *Lancet Infectious Diseases* 2 (2002): 11-17. However, later studies suggest that while there may be short term benefits from treating infections in heart disease with antibiotics, mid-term impacts are negligable. O'Connor *et al.*, "Azithromycin for the Secondary Prevention of Coronary Heart Disease Events."

27.   "Genetics of Coronary Heart Disease," WebMD, revised July 21, 2000 [online], http://my.webmd.com/content/article/2/1675_50290.htm [March 30, 2003].

Chapter 2 Guess What?...

1.   Dennis Carson, "An Infectious Origin of Extraskeletal Calcification," *Proceedings of the National Academy of Sciences (PNAS)* 95, no. 14 (July 7, 1998): 7846-47.

2.   "Astronauts Risk Kidney Stones," *BBC*, November 8, 2001 [online], http://news.bbc.co.uk/1/hi/health/1643632.stm [February 15, 2003]. Also, "Renal Stone Risk During Space Flight: Assessment and Countermeasure Validation," *NASA Fact Sheet*, July 2001 [online], http://www1.msfc.nasa.gov/NEWSROOM/background/facts/renal.html [February 15, 2003].

3.   "Ankylosing Spondylitis–Exams and Tests," WebMD [online], http://my.webmd.com/content/healthwise/10/2415.htm?lastselectedguid={5FE84E90-BC77-4056-A91C-9531713CA348} [March 15, 2003].

4.   Arteriosclerosis vs. atherosclerosis – See Introduction, endnote 1 to differentiate between these terms.

5.   T.W. Meade, "Cardiovascular Disease–Linking Pathology and Epidemiology," *International Journal of Epidemiology* 30, no.5 (October 2001): 1179-83.

6.   Daniel Q. Haney, "More Children Getting Adult Diabetes," *Associated Press*, April 13, 2003 [online], http://tory.news.yahoo.com/news?tmpl=story2&cid=541&ncid=751&e=6&u=/ap/0030413/ap_on_he_me/young_diabetes [April 10, 2003].

7.   Neal X. Chen and Sharon M. Moe, "Arterial Calcification in Diabetes," *Current Diabetes Reports* 3 (2003): 28-32 (February 1, 2003) Abstract [online], http://www.biomedcentral.com/1534-4827/3/28/abstract [April 10, 2003].

8. Peggy Lin, Lynne Goldberg, Tania Phillips, "Calciphylaxis," *Wounds* 14, no. 5 (2002): 205-10, Medscape [online], http://www.medscape.com/viewarticle/438054_5 [April 10, 2003].

9. "Salivary Stones," MayoClinic.com, January 12, 2002 [online], http://www.mayoclinic.com/invoke.cfm?id=HQ01323 [January 23, 2003].

10. Susan Kinder Haake, "Microbiology of Dental Plaque," Periodontics Information Center, University of California, Los Angeles School of Dentistry [online], http://www.dent.ucla.edu/pic/members/microbio/mdphome.html [March 29, 2003].

11. N. Çiftçioglu, D.S. McKay, E.O. Kajander, "Association Between Nanobacteria and Periodontal Disease," *Circulation* 108 (August 2003): 58-9.

12. "Cranial Calcification," Medline Plus Encyclopedia, National Institutes of Health January 10, 2003 [online], http://www.nlm.nih.gov/medlineplus/ency/imagepages/9228.htm [March 30, 2003].

13. E.M. Reiman, K. Chen, G.E. Alexander, R.J. Caselli, D. Bandy, A. Prouty, C. Burns, "Abnormalities in Regional Brain Activity in Young Adults at Genetic Risk for Late-onset Alzheimer's Disease," Abstract presentation at the 8th International Conference on Alzheimer's Disease and Related Disorders, Stockholm, 2002 [online], http://www.alz.washington.edu/PDF/azadc2.pdf [April 17, 2003].

14. "Alzheimer's Disease," Duke University Medical Center, Psychiatry and Behavioral Sciences [online], http://psychiatry.mc.duke.edu/CMRIS/ED/Alzheimers.htm [January 23, 2003].

15. "Clinical Guidelines for the Care of Patients with Tuberous Sclerosis Complex," Tuberous Sclerosis Association [online], http://www.tuberous-sclerosis.org/professionals/guidelines.shtml [January 23, 2003].

16. "Cancer Facts," National Institutes of Health [online], http://cis.nci.nih.gov/fact/5_6.htm [February 10, 2003].

17. "Mammogram Calcifications," Medline plus, National Institutes of Health [online], http://www.nlm.nih.gov/medlineplus/ency/article/002113.htm [January 23, 2003].

18. James H. Bedino, "Mycobacterium Tuberculosis: An In-depth Discussion for Embalmers Part 2," *Expanding Encyclopedia of Mortuary Practices* 637 (1999) [online], http://www.champion-newera.com/CHAMP.PDFS/encyclo637.pdf [April 26, 2003].

19. "Arthritis," National Center for Chronic Disease Prevention [online], http://www.cdc.gov/nccdphp/arthritis/index.htm [January 13, 2003].

20. "Ankylosing Spondylitis–Exams and Tests," WebMD [online], http://my.webmd.com/content/healthwise/10/2415.htm?lastselectedguid={5FE84E90-BC77-4056-A91C-9531713CA348} [March 15, 2003].

21. "Bone Spurs," spine-health.com [online], http://www.spine-health.com/topics/cd/spurs/spurs01.html) [February 10, 2003].

22. Robert Berkow (Editor-in-Chief), "Disorders of Muscles, Bursas, and Tendons," *The Merck Manual of Medical Information* Home Edition, Internet Edition, Chapter 55, 2000 [online], http://www.merck.com/mrkshared/mmanual_home/sec5/55.jsp [April 5, 2003].

23. "Bone Formation And Calcification In Cardiovascular Disease," National Institutes of Health, January 2, 2001 [online], http://grants2.nih.gov/grants/guide/rfa-files/RFA-HL-01-014.html [March 29, 2003]. Also, "New Evidence Connecting Cardiovascular Disease and Osteoporosis," National Institute of Arthritis and Musculoskeletal and Skin Diseases, NIAMS-NHLBI Working Group September 14-15, 1999 Bethesda, Maryland [online], http://www.niams.nih.gov/ne/reports/sci_wrk/1999/bnhrtsm.htm [April 3, 2003].

24. "Treatment for Vertigo May Provide Effective, Non-Surgical Relief for Meniere's Disease," News Release, American Academy of Otolaryngology Head and Neck Surgery September 21, 2002 [online], http://www.newswise.com/articles/2002/9/MENIERES.AAO.html [April 26, 2003]. Also: Ivy M. Alexander, "The Spin on Dizziness," *Yale Healthcare Newsletter* II, No 6. (1999) [online], http://www.yale.edu/yuhs/highlights/yhc/nov_dec99.pdf [April 10, 2003]. Also, information on calcification of inner ear stones provided in interview by the authors with Dr. Olavi Kajander April 25, 2003.

25. "What is Glaucoma?" Glaucoma Research Foundation [online], http://www.glaucoma.org/learn/ [January 15, 2003].

26. Teresa O'Sullivan, "Ocular Disorders," University of Washington School of Pharmacy [online], http://eduserv.hscer.washington.edu/pharmacy/pharm561/Week%2010/ocular.pdf [March 29, 2003].

27. "Macular Degeneration," Medline Plus Encyclopedia, National Institute of Health [online], http://www.nlm.nih.gov/medlineplus/ency/article/001000.htm#contentDescription [January 15, 2003].

28. "Drusen deposits vary in size and may exist in a variety of forms from soft to calcified." Quote from: "ARMD – The Disease. Age Related Macular Degeneration," Indiana University School of Optometry [online] http://www.opt.indiana.edu/clinics/pt_educ/armd/disease.htm [April 17, 2003].

29. Stephen B. Hanauer, "Overview of IBD Complications," Crohn's & Colitis Foundation of America, October 29, 1999 [online], http://www.ccfa.org/medcentral/library/compl/wkly1029.htm [March 29, 2003].

30. "Kidney Stones," National Kidney and Urologic Diseases Information Clearinghouse [online], http://www.niddk.nih.gov/health/kidney/pubs/stonadul/stonadul.htm#what. Also, "Nephrolithiasis," Medline Plus Encyclopedia, National Institutes of Health [online], http://www.nlm.nih.gov/medlineplus/ency/article/000458.htm [January 13, 2003].

31. Aijaz Ahmed, Emmet B. Keeffe, "Gallstones and Biliary Tract Disease," WebMD Scientific American Medicine February 28, 2003 [online], http://ww.medscape.com/viewarticle/449563_print [March 29, 2003].

32. "Addison's Disease," Medline Plus, National Institutes of Health [online], http://www.nlm.nih.gov/medlineplus/ency/article/000378.htm [January 15, 2003]. Also, telephone interview by the authors with Dr. Olavi Kajander, May 7, 2003 regarding kidney stones being a characteristic of Addison's disease.

33. "Hypoparathyroidism," Medline Plus Medical Encyclopedia, National Institutes of Health [online], http://www.nlm.nih.gov/medlineplus/ency/article/000385.htm [January 13, 2003].

34. Federico Guercini, "Prostatitis 2000 Symptoms," [online], http://www.prostatitis2000.org/eng/sintomatologia.htm [April 28, 2003].

35. "Kidney Stones," National Kidney and Urologic Diseases Information Clearinghouse [online], http://www.niddk.nih.gov/health/kidney/pubs/stonadul/stonadul.htm#what. Also, "Nephrolithiasis," Medline Plus Encyclopedia, National Institutes of Health [online], http://www.nlm.nih.gov/medlineplus/ency/article/000458.htm [January 13, 2003].

36. "Peyronie's Disease," National Kidney and Urologic Diseases Information Clearinghouse NIH Publication No. 01-3902 (May 1995, updated: September 2001) [online], http://www.niddk.nih.gov/health/urolog/pubs/peyronie/peyronie.htm [March 29, 2003].

37. Lisbeth Schjerling, Ebbe Kvist, Sven Grønvall Rasmussen & Anne Birthe Wåhlin, "Testicular Microlithiasis: the Necessity of Biopsy and Follow Up," Ugeskr Læger 164 (2002): 2041-45.

38. The protein is collagen. See: "Scleroderma," Arthritis Foundation [online], http://www.arthritis.org/conditions/DiseaseCenter/scleroderma.asp [January 17, 2003]. Also "Scleroderma," Amersham Health Encyclopedia [online], http://www.amershamhealth.com/medcyclopaedia/Volume%20III%201/scleroderma.asp [January 17, 2003].

39. G. C. Willis, "An Experimental Study of the Intimal Ground Substance in Atherosclerosis," *Canadian Medical Association Journal (CMAJ)* 69 (July 1953) [online], http://www.internetwks.com/pauling/study.html [April 3, 2003].

Chapter 3 How The "Sand In Our Motor Oil"...

1.   "Calcium," Chemical Elements.com [online], http://www.chemicalelements.com/elements/ca.html [January 1, 2003].

2.   Many physicians argue that we already have sufficient calcium in our bloodstream to make new bone without supplements being added. The problem, they say, is that in some cases as we age our bone making cells don't use it. "The body can only use so much calcium at a time. The rest is wasted," The Rhode Island Osteoporosis Program, Rhode Island Department of Health, Calcium and Vitamin D, updated August 21, 2002 [online], http://www.healthri.org/disease/osteoporosis/calcium.htm [March 29, 2003].

3.   Malcolm East, "Life, Death and Calcium," University of Southampton, March 2002, chembytes ezine, The Royal Society of Chemistry [online], http://www.chemsoc.org/chembytes/ezine/2002/east_mar02.htm [March 29, 2003].

4.   "Imbalances of calcium can lead to many health problems and excess calcium in nerve cells can cause their death." Quote from "Calcium," Cancerweb Dictionary, May 22, 1997 [online] http://cancerweb.ncl.ac.uk/cgi-bin/omd?calcium [January 15, 2003].

5.   "Apatite," Moh's Hardness Scale, Simon Fraser University Department of Archaeology [online], http://www.sfu.ca/archaeology/museum/rock_id/mohs%20scale.html [March 29, 2003].

6.   We attribute this term to Dr. Olavi Kajander who has used it in interviews with the authors.

7.   "Small Blood Vessels Big Role Found," *BBC* December 30, 2002 [online], http://news.bbc.co.uk/2/hi/health/2609469.stm [January 15, 2003]. Also, Matthew C.P. Glyn, John G. Lawrenson, and Barbara J. Ward, "A Rho-associated Kinase Mitigates Reperfusion-induced Change in the Shape of Cardiac Capillary Endothelial Cells in Situ," *Journal of Cardiovascular Research* 57, no. 1 (2003): 195-206, Abstract [online], http://www.elsevier.com/gej-ng/10/13/52/105/25/48/abstract.html [March 15, 2003].

8.   "Drug-free Way to Drop High Blood Pressure: Cut Calories, Add Exercise," Press Release, Report to the Annual Meeting of the American Heart Association, Chicago, September 24, 2001 [online], http://www.americanheart.org/presenter.jhtml?identifier=10993 [January 20, 2003].

9. "Calcium Scan Predicts Heart Attack Risk in Physically Fit People," *American Heart Association Journal Report,* January 3, 2001, http://www.americanheart.org/presenter.jhtml ?identifier=3292 [April 3, 2003]. The study authors Irwin M. Feuerstein, M.D., Michael P. Brazaitis, M.D., Mark A. Vaitkus, Ph.D., and William F. Barko, M.D., found that there is no apparent link between calcification and fitness level. "We were surprised by the high (calcium) scores in a group that was very physically fit and had undergone routine physical examinations," said Jerel M. Zoltick, M.D., a U.S. Army cardiologist and consultant with the Office of the Surgeon General.

10. Search results for the term "calcification" [online], http://www.intelihealth.com [April 17, 2003].

11. For example, when a patient asked about calcification of the optic nerve, known as Drusen, the advising physician noted: "Unfortunately, I know of no treatment for this when it happens." Don Carl Bienfang, "Ask The Expert," Intellihealth October 22, 2002 [online], http://www.intelihealth.com/IH/ihtIH?d=dmtATD&c =356533&p=~br,IHW|~st,24479|~r, WSIHW000|~b,*| [April 17, 2003]. Responses by experts regarding coronary artery calcification and spinal stenosis also had no suggestions other than surgery for removing calcium deposits. See http://www.intelihealth.com/IH/ihtIH?d=dmtATD&c= 328362&p=~br,IHW|~st,24479|~r, WSIHW000|~b,*| and http://www.intelihealth.com/IH/ ihtIH?d=dmtATD&c=331924&p=~br,IHW| ~st,24479|~r,WSIHW000|~b,*| [April 17, 2003].

12. Johns Hopkins Arthritis Radiology Rounds states that "the cause of calcinosis cutis is unknown." *Radiology Rounds*, Round 7 [online], http://www.hopkins-arthritis.som.jhmi.edu/radrds/radiology_7/7_radrds_diagnosis.html [April 17, 2003].

13. A good summary of contemporary thinking on this is: Paul W. Ewald, *Plague Time: How Stealth Infections Cause Cancers, Heart Disease and Other Deadly Ailments* (New York: Anchor Books, 2002).

14. Beth Israel Deaconess Medical Center Website [online], http://www.bidmc.harvard.edu/radiology/heartscan/intro.html [January 15, 2003]. Note that this facility trains Harvard Medical School doctors.

15. Website of the American Heart Association [online], http://www.heartcenteronline.com/myheartdr/common/rtprn_rev.cfm? filename=&ARTID=191 [December 18, 2002].

16. Word search for "calcification" using www.google.com [September 15, 2003].

17. Ibid. Word search using "cause of calcification."

18. Martin Bendszus, "Brain Damage After Surgical and Angiographic Heart Procedures," *Geriatric Times* IV , issue 1 (January/February 2003) [online], http://www.geriatrictimes.com/g030231.html [March 29, 2003].

19. Ron Winslow, "New Stents a Boon for Patients May Affect Rising Health Costs," *Wall Street Journal* (December 24, 2002), p.1.

20. Ibid.

21. "Extracorporeal Shock Wave Lithotripsy for the Treatment of Gallstones, Pancreatic Stones and Bile Duct Stones," *The Regence Group Medical Policy Manual*, approved date 05/07/2002 [online], http://www.regence.com/trgmedpol/surgery/sur81.html [January 27, 2003]; and "Kidney Stones Frequently Asked Questions," Your Medical Source [online], http://yourmedicalsource.com/library/kidneystones/KS_faq.html [January 27, 2003].

22. The role of clotting in calcification is presently under investigation by a team led by Dr. Olavi Kajander at NanobacLabs Research Institute in Tampa, Florida. Interview by the authors with Dr. Kajander April 26, 2003.

23. This is the emerging theory of atherogenesis referred to later in the book, as developed under the leadership of Dr. Gary Mezo at NanobacLabs Research Institute.

24. A description of the body's self-destructive response to injury in the artery is found at: M. R. (Pete) Hayden, "Atherosclerosis and Plaque Angiogenesis: a Malignant Transformation," Pathology and Clinical Classification of Vulnerable Plaque, May 20, 2001 [online], http://www.vp.org/ResourceCenter/Pete_Hayden_Angiogenesis.html [March 29, 2003].

25. Daniel Q. Haney "Vulnerable Plaque, the Latest in Heart Disease?" *Associated Press*, January 11, 1999 [online], http://www.canoe.com/Health9901/11_heart.html. "By the time you see an irregularity on the angiogram, the first little 25 per cent narrowing, over 85 per cent of the rest of the arteries are atherosclerotic. It's all hidden." Dr. Steven Nissen, Cleveland Clinic.

26. "Coronary Artery Disease," The Harvard Medical School Family Health Guide, New York Simon & Schuster, 1999, updated 2003 [online], http://www.health.harvard.edu/fhg/fhgupdate/K/K2.shtml [April 14, 2003].

27. "Toshiba Receives FDA Clearance On Cardiac Functional Analysis Package For The Aquilion™16 Multislice Ct Scanner," Tustin, California, December 18, 2002 [online], http://www.medical.toshiba.com/news/pressreleases/121802-434.htm [April 17, 2003].

Chapter 4 The Nano Detectives

1. A description of how the polio vaccine is prepared is found in: "The Withdrawal of an Oral Polio Vaccine: Analysis of Events and Implications. A Report by the Chief Medical Officer CMO OPV," Report June 2002, Department of Health, U.K. [online], http://www.doh.gov.uk/cmo/opvreport/opvrepjun02.pdf [March 30, 2003].

2. Christine Stencel, Cory Arberg, "More Data Needed to Determine if Contaminated Polio Vaccine From 1955-1963 Causes Cancer in Adults Today," National Academies, Press Release Oct. 22, 2002 [online], http://www4.nas.edu/news.nsf/isbn/0309086108?OpenDocument [January 18, 2003].

3. Professor Carson is now Director of the Sam and Rose Stein Institute for Research on Aging at University of California, San Diego.

4. Joel B. Baseman, Joseph G. Tully, "Mycoplasmas: Sophisticated, Reemerging, and Burdened by Their Notoriety," *Emerging Infectious Diseases* 3, No.1 (January-March 1997): 21-32.

5. Interview by the authors with E. Olavi Kajander on April 23, 2003.

6. United States Patent Office. United States Patent 5,135,851

7. Interview by the authors with E. Olavi Kajander, October 15, 2002.

8. "Diagnosis of mycoplasma infections...has had a troubling history... With the application of molecular genetic technology, new methods have been developed such as DNA fingerprinting..." Quote from David MacKenzie, "Epidemiology and Control of Emerging Strains of Poultry Respiratory Disease Agents," Northeastern Regional Association of State Agricultural Experiment Station Directors, November 10, 2002 [online], http://www.lgu.umd.edu/project/outline.cfm?trackID=10#top [April 10, 2003].

9. Ibid.

10. T.G. Harrison, N. Doshi, "Serological Evidence of Bartonella spp. Infection in the UK," *Epidemiol Infect* 123, no.2 (Oct. 1999): 233-40.

11. Robert Kunzig, "The Unbearably Unstoppable Neutrino," *Discover Magazine* 22, no. 8 (August 2001): 40.

12. "Size Limits of Very Small Microorganisms," Proceedings of a Workshop October 22-23, 1998, Washington, D.C., Panel 2, Space Studies Board, National Academy of Sciences [online], http://www7.nationalacademies.org/ssb/nanopanel2Kajander.html [March 30, 2003].

13.   N. Çiftçioglu, M. A. Miller-Hjelle, J. T. Hjelle, and E. O. Kajander, "Inhibition of Nanobacteria by Antimicrobial Drugs as Measured by a Modified Microdilution Method," *Antimicrobial Agents and Chemotherapy* 46, no. 7 (July 2002): 2077-86 [online], http://aac.asm.org/cgi/content/full/46/7/2077?maxtoshow=&HITS=10&hits=10&RESULTFORMAT=&titleabstract=nanobacteria&searchid=1043171003292_7860&stored_search=&FIRSTINDEX=0&search_url=http%3A%2F%2Fjournals.asm.org%2Fcgi%2Fsearch [January 21, 2003].

Chapter 5 Challenging The Definition Of Life

1.   "Cold Fusion Farewell," *New Scientist* 157, no. 2126 (21 March 1998): 23.

2.   L. G. Puskás *et al.*, "Detection of *Nanobacterium sanguineum* in Human Atherosclerotic Plaques," Hungarian Academy of Science, DNA-Chip Laboratory, Departments of Pathology, Pharmacology, and Pharmacotherapy, University of Szeged, Hungary. This paper was submitted to journals but never published. In interviews with the authors, Drs. Kajander and Çiftçioglu credited him with the discovery. Mayo Clinic researchers Rasmussen *et al.* (see next note) refer indirectly to his work in their research paper that duplicated some of his findings.

3.   Todd E. Rasmussen, Brenda L. Kirkland, Jon Charlesworth, George P. Rodgers, Sandra R. Severson, Jeri Rodgers, Robert L. Folk, Virginia M. Miller, "Electron Microscope and Immunological Evidence of Nanobacterial-like Structures in Calcified Carotid Arteries, Aortic Aneurysms and Cardiac Valves," *Journal of the American College of Cardiology (JACC)* 39, issue 5 (6 March 2002): Supplement A.

4.   J. T. Hjelle, M. A. Miller-Hjelle, I. R. Poxton, O. Kajander, N. Çiftçioglu, M. L. Jones, R. C. Caughey, R. Brown, P. D. Millikin, F. S. Darras, "Endotoxin and Nanobacteria in Polycystic Kidney Disease," *Kidney International* 57 (2000): 2360-74.

5.   The term "nannobacteria" (with two n's) was first used in scientific literature by Richard Y. Morita, "Bioavailibility of Energy and Starvation Survival in Nature," *Canadian Journal of Microbiology* 34 (1988): 436-41. Also: Robert L. Folk, "Nanobacteria: Surely Not Figments, But What Under Heaven Are They?" *Natural Science* 1, Article 3 (1997) [online], http://naturalscience.com/ns/articles/01-03/ns_folk.html [January 25, 2003].

6.   Robert L. Folk, "Nanobacteria: Surely Not Figments, But What Under Heaven Are They?" *Natural Science.*

7.   D. S. McKay, E. K. Gibson Jr., K. L. Thomas-Keprta, H. Vali, C. S. Romanek, S. J. Clemett, X. D. F. Chillier, C. R. Maechling, R.

N. Zare, "Search for Past Life on Mars: Possible Relic Biogenic Activity in Martian Meteorite ALH84001," *Science* 273, no. 5277 (August 16, 1996): 924-30.

8. N. Boyce, "The Martians in Your Kidneys," *New Scientist* 163, issue 2200 (August 21, 1999): 32.

9. Philippa J.R. Uwins, Richard I. Webb, Anthony P. Taylor, "Novel Nano-Organisms From Australian Sandstone," *American Mineralogist* 83 (1998): 1541-50 [online], http://www.microscopy-uk.org.uk/nanobes/nanobes.pdf [January 20, 2003]. See also Dr. Uwins' website at http://www.uq.edu.au/nanoworld/uwins.html [January 20, 2003].

10. Ibid.

11. Harald Huber, Michael J. Hohn, Reinhard Rachel, Tanja Fuchs, Verena C. Wimmer & Karl O. Stetter, "A New Phylum of Archaea Represented by a Nanosized Hyperthermophilic Symbiont," *Nature* 417 (May 02, 2002): 63-67 [online], http://www.nature.com/cgi-taf/DynaPage.taf?file=/nature/journal/v417/n6884/full/417063a_r.html [January 20, 2003].

12. Diversa Corporation, through its collaboration with the laboratory of Professor Karl Stetter of the University of Regensburg and Celera Genomics, an Applera Corporation business, announced that it completed the sequencing and annotation of the smallest archaeal genome discovered to date, *Nanoarchaeum equitans*. Stephen Hart, "Minimalist Life," *Astrobiology Magazine* (18 December 2002).

13. Dennis Carson, "An Infectious Origin of Extraskeletal Calcification," *Proceedings of the National Academy of Sciences* 95 (1998): 7846-47.

14. Interview by the authors with Olavi Kajander, October 15, 2002. Also, N. Ciftcioglu, E. O. Kajander, "Interaction of Nanobacteria with Cultured Mammalian Cells," *Pathophysiology* 4 (1998): 259-70. The total definition is far more complex, as we see in the rest of this chapter.

15. E. Olavi Kajander and Neva Çiftçioglu, "Nanobacteria: An Alternative Mechanism for Pathogenic Intra- and Extracellular Calcification and Stone Formation," *Proceedings of the National Academy of Sciences (PNAS) USA* 95, issue 14 (1998): 8274-79.

16. Charles F. A. Bryce, "Alternative View on the Putative Organism, *Nanobacterium sanguineum*," Braids Education Consultants, Edinburgh EH10 6NZ, Scotland (UNDATED) [online], http://www.heartfixer.com/Nanobacterium-Report.htm [January 23, 2003].

17. Kenneth Nealson, "Panel 2 Discussion Summarized by K. Nealson," Size Limits of Very Small Microorganisms, Proceed-

ings of a Workshop October 22-23, 1998, Washington, D.C., Space Studies Board, National Academy of Sciences [online], http://www7.nationalacademies.org/ssb/nanopanel2.html [March 30, 2003].

18. E. Olavi Kajander, Mikael Björklund, and Neva Çiftçioglu, "Suggestions from Observations on Nanobacteria Isolated from Blood," Panel 2 (Continued) Abstract, Size Limits of Very Small Microorganisms, Proceedings of a Workshop October 22-23, 1998, Washington, D.C., Space Studies Board, National Academy of Sciences [online], http://www7.nationalacademies.org/ssb/nanopanel2Kajander.html [March 30, 2003].

19. Interview by the authors with Olavi Kajander October 16, 2002.

20. Note from Gary Mezo to the authors May 5, 2003.

21. Jeffrey G. Lawrence, "Gene Transfer and Minimal Genome Size," Panel 1, Size Limits of Very Small Microorganisms, Proceedings of a Workshop October 22-23, 1998, Washington, D.C., Space Studies Board, National Academy of Sciences [online], http://www7.nationalacademies.org/ssb/nanopanel1lawrence.html [April 30, 2003].

22. Olavi Kajander, "Alleged Nanobacteria Exist and Participate in Calcification of Arterial Plaque, Response to November 2002 issue having Elmer M. Cranton's letter 'Alleged Nanobacteria Do Not Cause Calcification of Arterial Plaque'," Nanobac Oy website [online], http://www.nanobac.com/press.html [January 20, 2003]. See also discussion paper with that comparison: Peter B. Moore, "A Biophysical Chemist's Thoughts on Cell Size," Size Limits of Very Small Microorganisms, Proceedings of a Workshop October 22-23, 1998, Washington, D.C., Panel 1, Space Studies Board, National Academy of Sciences [online], http://www7.nationalacademies.org/ssb/nanopanel1moore.html [March 20, 2003].

23. Alison Abbott, "Battle Lines Drawn Between 'Nanobacteria' Researchers," *Nature* 401 (September 9, 1999): 105.

24. U.S. patent 5,135,851.

25. Email from Matti Uusitupa Rector, University of Kuopio, Finland, to Douglas Mulhall, November 21, 2002.

26. The complaint was later filed with the Central Science Ethics Committee of Finland (approx. translation of title from Finnish), where it was also rejected. Interview by the authors with E. Olavi Kajander, April 23, 2003.

27. John O. Cisar, De-Qi Xu, John Thompson, William Swaim, Lan Hu, Dennis J. Kopecko, "An Alternative Interpretation of Nanobacteria-induced Biomineralization," *Proceedings of the National Academy of Sciences* 97 (10 October 2000): 11511-15.

28. Open Session Minutes, Food and Drug Administration, Center for Biologics Evaluation and Research, Vaccines and Biological Products Advisory Committee, Bethesda Maryland, November 18, 2002 [online], http://www.fda.gov/ohrms/dockets/ac/02/transcripts/3906T1.doc, 14 [April 30, 2003]. Note: Kajander's name was misspelled in the minutes as "Pejander."

29. E. Olavi Kajander, Neva Çiftçioglu, Katja M. Aho, "Detection of Nanobacteria in Viral Vaccines," Proceedings of the American Society for Microbiology, 101 General Meeting, Orlando, May 20-24, 2001 [online], http://www.asmusa.org/memonly/abstracts/AbstractView.asp?AbstractID= 50191 [March 30, 2003].

30. Open Session Minutes, Food and Drug Administration, transcript, p. 14.

31. Cisar et al., "An Alternative Interpretation of Nanobacteria-induced Biomineralization," PNAS 97 (Oct. 10, 2000).

32. Correspondence from Dr. Kopecko to the authors June 6, 2003.

33. Open Session Minutes, Food and Drug Administration, transcript, p. 14.

34. Cisar et al., "An Alternative Interpretation of Nanobacteria-induced Biomineralization." The FDA's website also refers to J. O. Cisar, D. Q. Xu, J. Thompson, W. Swaim, L. Hu, D. J. Kopecko, "Absence of nanobacteria in human saliva and dental plaque," Dental Research 79 (Special Issue 2000): 2231.

35. E. Olavi Kajander, "Alleged Nanobacteria Exist and Participate in Calcification of Arterial Plaque, Response to November 2002 issue having Elmer M. Cranton's letter 'Alleged Nanobacteria Do Not Cause Calcification of Arterial Plaque'," Nanobac Oy website [online], http://www.nanobac.com/press.html [January 20, 2003].

36. Ibid.

37. Correspondence from Dr. Kopecko to the authors June 6, 2003 and from Dr. Kajander to the authors June 19, 2003.

38. Correspondence from Dr. Kajander to the authors June 19, 2003.

39. Rasmussen et al., "Electron Microscopic and Immunological Evidence of Nanobacterial-Like Structures," JACC 39, issue 5 (6 March 2002): Supplement A.

40. Puskás wrote a paper on this that was submitted to various journals but was never published. However, in interviews with the authors, Kajander and Çiftçioglu both credited him with the discovery.

41. A. Sommer, J. Christoffersen, M. R. Christoffersen "New Evidence Indicating that Initial Mineralization of Nanobacteria In-

volves an Active Process," submission in preparation, email to the authors, May 19, 2003.

42. Katja Aho, E. Olavi Kajander, "Pitfalls in the Detection of Novel Nanoorganisms," Letters to the Editor, *Journal of Clinical Microbiology* 41, 7 (Jul. 2003): 3460-61. This letter compares the characteristics of nanobacteria with other pathogens, such as viruses and conventionally known bacteria, presenting data that nanobacteria are a unique life form. The table is excerpted in this book as "How to tell *Nanobacterium sanguineum*" (see Figure 8).

43. "People who received polio vaccine between 1954 and 1962 may have received a dose that contained SV40. As many as 10 to 30 million persons in the U.S. could have received SV40-contaminated injectable polio vaccine." "Concerns About Vaccine Contamination," Center for Disease Control website [online], http://www.cdc.gov/nip/vacsafe/concerns/gen/contamination.htm [January 26, 2003].

44. "…we have never noticed formation of biofilm on plastic surfaces." Michel Drancourt, Véronique Jacomo, Hubert Lépidi, Eric Lechevallier, Vincent Grisoni, Christian Coulange, Edith Ragni, Claude Alasia, Bertrand Dussol, Yvon Berland, Didier Raoult, "Attempted Isolation of Nanobacterium sp. Microorganisms from Upper Urinary Tract Stones," *Journal of Clinical Microbiology* 41, no. 1 (January 2003): 368-72, Abstract [online], http://jcm.asm.org/cgi/content/abstract/41/1/368 [February 15, 2003].

45. Telephone interview by the authors with Neva Çiftçioglu, January 15, 2003.

46. "Kidney Stones in Adults," National Kidney and Urologic Disease Clearinghouse, National Institutes of Health [online], http://www.niddk.nih.gov/health/kidney/pubs/stonadul/stonadul.htm#who [March 27, 2003].

47. Ibid.

48. Ibid.

49. "What Causes Kidney Stones?" UC Davis Health System Medical Conditions A-Z list 2001 [online], http://www.ucdmc.ucdavis.edu/ucdhs/health/a-z/81kidneystones/doc81causes.html [April 17, 2003].

50. E. Olavi Kajander and Neva Çiftçioglu, "Nanobacteria: An Alternative Mechanism for Pathogenic Intra- and Extracellular Calcification and Stone Formation," *Proceedings of the National Academy of Sciences (PNAS) USA* 95, issue 14 (1998): 8274-79.

51. Ibid.

52. "About PKD," The PKD Foundation [online], http://www.pkdcure.org/aboutPkd.htm [March 29, 2003].

53. J. T. Hjelle *et al.*, "Endotoxins and Nanobacteria in Polycystic Kidney Disease," *Kidney International* 57 (2000): 2360-74.

54. Ibid.

55. The study "Pathogenesis Of Calcium Nephrolithiasis," directed by Fredric Coe, has been awarded financing by the NIH for fiscal years 1998-2002, see [online], http://grants2.nih.gov/grants/award/state/fy2000.illinois.txt [April 10, 2003]. Also, NIH, PO 1 DK 56788, Pathogenesis and Treatment of Calcium Nephrolithiasis. F. L. Coe, Principal Investigator. Project 3 - Mechanism of Stone Formation in the Rat and Core C - Genetic Hypercalciuric Stone Forming Rats. D. A. Bushinsky, Principal Investigator [online], http://www.urmc.rochester.edu/medicine/AnnualRpt/EndoFac.pdf [April 10, 2003]. Coe emphasized in an email message to the authors June 23, 2003 that his research has nothing to do with research by the scientists who are working on nanobacteria. However, we have included reference to Coe's work here due to the apparent similarities between the calcium phosphate found in his new studies and the material found by nanobacterial researchers in kidney stones.

56. Andrew P. Evan, James E. Lingerman, Fredric L. Coe, Joan H. Parks, Sharon B. Bledsoe, Youzhi Shao, Andre J. Sommer, Ryan F. Paterson, Ramsay L. Kuo, Marc Grynpas, "Randall's Plaque of Patients with Nephrolithiasis Begins in Basement Membranes of Thin Loops of Henle," *Journal of Clinical Investigation* 111 (2003): 607-16.

57. Mayo Clinic posting for researchers [online], http://www.mayo.edu/research/postdoc/lieske1.html [March 30, 2003].

58. J. T. Hjelle *et al.*, "Endotoxins and Nanobacteria in Polycystic Kidney Disease," *Kidney International* 57 (2000): 2360-74.

59. Katja Aho, E. Olavi Kajander, "Pitfalls in the Detection of Novel Nanoorganisms," Letters to the Editor, *Journal of Clinical Microbiology* 41, 7 (Jul 2003): 3460-61. This letter compares the characteristics of nanobacteria with other pathogens, such as viruses and conventionally known bacteria, presenting data that nanobacteria are a unique life form. The table is excerpted in this book as "How to tell *Nanobacterium sanguineum*" (see Figure 8).

60. Ibid.

61. "Just as physicists recognize light either as electromagnetic waves or as particulate photons, depending on the context, so biologists can profitably regard viruses both as exceptionally simple microbes and as exceptionally complex chemicals." R. Dulbecco and H. S. Ginsberg, *Virology* (1980) (originally published as a section of *Microbiology*, 3rd. ed., by Davis *et al.*, Harper and Row, Hagerstown, MD); p. 855 [online], http://web.uct.ac.za/microbiology/tutorial/molechis.htm [March 18, 2003].

Chapter 6 Seeds Of Destruction?

1. Rasmussen *et al.*, "Electron Microscope and Immunological Evidence of Nanobacterial-like Structures," *JACC* 39, issue 5 (6 March 2002): Supplement A.

2. Benedict S. Maniscalco, "Shouldering the Risk Burden: Infection, Atherosclerosis, and the Vascular Endothelium," *Circulation* 107 (Mar 2003): 74. Also, Hyo-Chun Yoon, Aletha M. Emerick, Jennifer A. Hill, David W. Gjertson, and Jonathan G. Goldin, "Calcium Begets Calcium: Progression of Coronary Artery Calcification in Asymptomatic Subjects," *Radiology* 224 (2002): 236-41.

3. E. Olavi Kajander, M. Bjorklund, N. Çiftçioglu, "Nanobacteria and Man" in *Enigmatic Microorganisms and Life in Extreme Environments*, edited by J. Seckbach (Dordrecht, Netherlands: Kluwer Academic Publishers, 1999), 195-203. Also, interview between Dr. Olavi Kajander and the authors on April 22, 2003.

4. K. Ackerman, I. Kuronen, O. Kajander, "Scanning Electron Microscopy of Nanobacteria-Novel Biofilm Producing Organisms in Blood," *Scanning* 15, III (1993).

5. "Identification of Bacterial Genes and Cell Structure(s) Inducing $CaCO_3$ Precipitation," Bioreinforce Project, EC Programme "Energy, Environment and Sustainable Development" [online], http://www.ub.es/rpat/bioreinforce/ReportWeb.PDF [April 17, 2003].

6. E. Olavi Kajander, M. Bjorklund, N. Çiftçioglu, "Nanobacteria and Man." Also interview between the authors and Dr. Kajander on April 22, 2003.

7. The role of nanobacteria in formation of kidney stones is summarized in: E. Olavi Kajander, Neva Çiftçioglu, Katja Aho, Enrique Garcia-Cuerpo, "Characteristics of Nanobacteria and Their Possible Role in Stone Formation," Invited Editorial, *Urological Research* 31, 2 (Jun. 2003): 47-54, Abstract pre-published April 2003 [online], http://link.springer.de/link/service/journals/00240/contents/03/00304/ [April 30, 2003]. For other research on formation of kidney stones due to calcification see; Andrew P. Evan, James E. Lingerman, Fredric L. Coe, Joan H. Parks, Sharon B. Bledsoe, Youzhi Shao, Andre J. Sommer, Ryan F. Paterson, Ramsay L. Kuo, Marc Grynpas, "Randall's Plaque of Patients with Nephrolithiasis Begins in Basement Membranes of Thin Loops of Henle," *Journal of Clinical Investigation* 111 (2003): 607-16.

8. See also E.O. Kajander, K.M. Aho, B.S. Maniscalco, G.S. Mezo, "The Pathogenesis of Vascular Calcification, New Clinical Diagnostic Markers and a New Curative Nanobiotic Treatment for

Reversing Atherosclerosis in Humans," Poster session, Tampere, Finland, February 21, 2003.

9. Neva Çiftçioglu, E. Olavi Kajander, "Interaction of Nanobacteria with Cultured Mammalian Cells," *Pathophysiology* 4 (1998): 258-70.

10. The discoveries of how nanobacteria act in atherosclerosis and how to get rid of them have a few turns to them. In 1998, Prof. Dennis Carson published his PNAS commentary "An Infectious Origin of Extraskeletal Calcification," *Proceedings of the National Academy of Sciences (PNAS)* that surmised, based on data from Kajander, Çiftçioglu, and others, that nanobacteria and other pathogens may play a role in the body's inflammatory response to atherosclerotic vascular damage. Around 1999 László Puskás detected nanobacteria in atherosclerotic plaque. By then, the use of EDTA for dissolving calcium shells and the use of tetracycline for killing nanobacteria *in vitro* had been discovered and applied by Kajander and Çiftçioglu since the early 1990s, and published, for example, in "A New Potential Threat in Antigen and Antibody Products: Nanobacteria," Neva Çiftçioglu, Ilpo Kuronen, Kari Akerman, Erkki Hiltunen, Jukka Laukkanen and E. Olavi Kajander, *Vaccines 97*, Brown & al ed., (New York, Cold Spring Harbor Laboratory Press, 1997). On the other hand, the discovery and development of how to effectively get rid of nanobacteria in atherosclerosis *in vivo* (i.e. in human subjects) was Gary Mezo's. He used the then-known EDTA and tetracycline combination with other chemicals in a special formula and sequence that made the combination work effectively in the human metabolism. This new combination succeeded, according to cardiologists interviewed for this book and the clinical trial supervised by Dr. Benedict Maniscalco (paper in submission), to measurably reverse the clinical signs of atherosclerosis in patients. Theorization about the pathophysiological role of nanobacteria has emerged from the confluence of those discoveries. Dr. Mezo has indicated to the authors that he plays the leading role in developing this "unifying theory of atherogenesis." Dr. Çiftçioglu adds that, as with most theories, Dr. Mezo's draws from earlier published works, in this case by those done by Carson, Çiftçioglu, Kajander, and others.

11. Philippe Brunet, Yvon Berland, "Water Quality Complications of Haemodialysis," *Nephrology Dialysis Transplantation* 15 (2000): 578-80.

12. E.B. Breitschwerdt, Sushama Sontakke, Allen Cannedy, Susan I. Hancock, Julie M. Bradley, "Infection with *Bartonella Weissii* and Detection of Nanobacterium Antigens in a North Carolina Beef Herd," *Journal of Clinical Microbiology* 39 (2001): 879-82.

13. Neva Çiftçioglu, "Risk for Nanobacteria in Gamma Globulin Preparations," 102nd General Meeting of the American Society

for Microbiology, Salt Lake City, Utah, May 19-23, 2002, (Session 165, Paper Y-10) [online], http://www.asmusa.org/pcsrc/gm2002/1935.htm [March 30, 2003]. For additional supporting data see next endnote.

14. E. Olavi Kajander, Neva Çiftçioglu, Katja M. Aho, "Detection of Nanobacteria in Viral Vaccines," Proceedings of the American Society for Microbiology, 101 General Meeting, Orlando, May 20-24, 2001 [online], http://www.asmusa.org/memonly/abstracts/AbstractView.asp?AbstractID=50191 [March 30, 2003]. Also, M. Holmberg, "Prevalence of Human Anti-Nanobacteria Antibodies Suggest Possible Zoonosis," abstract, International Nanobacteria Minisymposium, Kuopio March 8, 2001 [online], http://www.nanobac.com/nbminisymp080301/page10.html [March 30, 2003].

Chapter 7 The Entrepreneurial Practitioner

1. Dr. Benedict Maniscalco, M.D., F.A.C.C. Personal interview with the authors, October 16, 2002.

2. Jennifer Thomas, "Is There a Doctor in the House?" *HealthScout News*, Healthfinder [online], http://www.health-finder.gov/news/newsstory.asp? docID=506980 [March 3, 2003].

3. "Nutraceuticals (often referred to as phytochemicals or functional foods) are natural, bioactive chemical compounds that have health promoting, disease preventing or medicinal properties." The Nutraceutical Institute [online], http://foodsci.rutgers.edu/nci/#what [January 21, 2003].

4. Whole books have been written about chelation. There is evidence on both sides about the success of the various types of chelation. Many patients and doctors swear by it. Other physicians say that it is dangerous. While we generally explain the role of EDTA as a sequestering agent for the purposes of describing the nanobiotic therapies of Nanobac Pharmaceuticals, we as authors do not consider ourselves qualified to have a position on what is commonly referred to as "chelation." For that reason we have mentioned both sides of the discussion without comment. We also await the outcome of the $30 million National Institutes of Health study on this topic.

5. EDTA has been used for decades, sometimes with measurable results, other times with disputed ones. Its lead-removing properties have been known for many years. It has been the treatment of choice for heavy metal toxicity. D. O. Shiels, D. L. G. Thomas, and E. Kearley, "Treatment of Lead Poisoning by Edathamil Calcium-Disodium," *AMA Arch. Indust. Health* 13 (1956), 489, 497. It has been a generic prescription-only medicine since the 1970's and is rated by the FDA as GRAS (Generally Recognized

As Safe). For a summary of other applications of EDTA, see: "Questions & Answers: The NIH Trial of EDTA Chelation Therapy for Coronary Artery Disease," National Center for Complementary Medicine, August 7, 2002 [online], http://nccam.nih.gov/news/2002/chelation/q-and-a.htm [March 30, 2003].

6.   Marsha Cohen, "Pharmacy Compounding," excerpted from Chapter VIII, "Preparation of Drugs by a Pharmacy," *Pharmacy Law for California Pharmacists*, 4th ed., by William L. Marcus and Marsha N. Cohen (2002) [online], http://www.uchastings.edu/cohen/gmos.htm [March 30, 2003].

7.   There are conflicting reports on chelation and kidney damage. A 2003 study found that EDTA chelation therapy may actually improve kidney function in some cases. See J.-L. Lin, D.-T. Lin-Tan, K.-H. Hsu, C.-C Yu, "Environmental Lead Exposure and Progression of Chronic Renal Diseases in Patients without Diabetes," *New England Journal of Medicine* 348 (Jan. 23, 2003): 277-86. However, the American Cancer Society and other authorities say that chelation has the "potential" to cause kidney damage, although documentation on this claim is disputed. "Chelation," American Cancer Society Guide to Complementary and Alternative Methods [online], http://www.cancer.org/docroot/ETO/content/ETO_5_3X_Chelation_Therapy.asp?sitearea=ETO [April 10, 2003].

8.   In a note to the authors May 5, 2003, Dr. Mezo indicated that he measured creatinine (a waste product from the body's use of protein) and BUN (blood urea nitrogen from the breakdown of blood, muscle and protein). He also conducted Liver Function Studies on patients.

9.   Note from Gary Mezo to the authors May 5, 2003.

Chapter 8 How Do I Know If I Have Them?

1.   The original tests for detecting nanobacteria were developed by Drs. Kajander and Çiftçioglu, then licensed to Nanobac Oy laboratories in Finland, which was subsequently acquired by Nanobac Pharmaceuticals (formerly NanobacLabs) in Tampa, Florida.

2.   Martin Holmberg, "Prevalence of Human Anti-Nanobacteria Antibodies Suggest Possible Zoonosis," Abstract Nanobacteria Minisymposium Kuopio 2002 [online], http://www.nanobac.com/nbminisymp080301/page10.html [April 10, 2003].

3.   According to Drs. Olavi Kajander, Benedict Maniscalco, and Gary Mezo, 100 percent of their respective heart disease patients who

were tested for nanobacteria came up positive. Kajander maintains that "if you find nanobacteria in 15 per cent of the general population (as a Finnish study did), then find that close to 100 percent of heart disease patients test positive, then that is significant." Interviews with Gary Mezo and Olavi Kajander, April 25, 2003, and with Benedict Maniscalco, March 16, 2003.

4. Excerpt from the Nanobac Pharmaceuticals website [online], http://www.NanobacLabs.com/NanobacLabs-nanobacteria-testing.asp [January 1, 2003]:

"The NanobacTEST-U/A rapid ELISA test is an inexpensive on-the-spot urine test that checks for the presence of nanobacteria, with visual results in minutes! The Nanobac-TEST-U/A rapid urine screening test tells the physician if you have active nanobacterial antigen from infection by detecting the presence of live uncalcified nanobacteria in your urine at the time of the test.

"The NanobacTEST-U/A rapid urine screening test is similar in operation to an OTC home urine pregnancy test, i.e.: two drops of urine are placed in the test well, a red "Control" stripe will signify proper function of the test, and if the urine is positive for *Nanobacterium sanguineum* Antigen, a red stripe in the "Test" section will be visible.

"The NanobacTEST-S is a serum blood test that checks for both nanobacterial antigen and antibodies in your blood. The NanobacTEST-S provides the physician with valuable information such as:

1.) Are there live uncalcified nanobacteria in the blood at the time of the test? If nanobacteria are present, how severe is the infection?

2.) Has the patient developed Antibodies to the Nanobacterial LPS Biofilm? Quantitatively and qualitatively, what is the patient's immune response to the nanobacterial infection?"

5. "CAT Scan," *Medline plus*, National Institutes of Health [online], http://www.nlm.nih.gov/medlineplus/ency/article/003330.htm [March 30, 2003].

6. "Thoracic CT," *Medline plus*, National Institutes of Health [online], http://www.nlm.nih.gov/medlineplus/ency/article/003788.htm [January 21, 2003]

Chapter 9 Ungumming Our Machinery

1. Nanobac Pharmaceuticals (previously NanobacLabs) is the first company to develop a nanobiotic treatment. The company has the most clinical experience and counts among its research col-

laborators Dr. Olavi Kajander, the discoverer who patented *Nanobacterium sanguineum*, and Dr. Neva Çiftçioglu, the co-developer of tests for detecting it. It is the sole licensee of the original tests developed by Nanobac Oy in Finland for detecting such nanobacteria. The company is led by the developer of the nanobiotic treatment, Dr. Gary Mezo. In June of 2003, American Enterprise Corporation acquired controlling interest in NanobacLabs through a share swap. The companies then adopted the name Nanobac Pharmaceuticals. The information presented here about the treatment is gleaned from their literature and from interviews with Drs. Kajander, Çiftçioglu, Mezo, and participating physicians. At least one other group has begun to develop and apply treatments for nanobacterial infections. As of the date of writing of this book, that later-developed treatment has not to the authors' knowledge resulted in the presentation of clinical findings, and for that reason we do not cover it here.

2. Shiels *et al.*, "Treatment of Lead Poisoning By Edathamil Calcium-Disodium." Also, "Questions & Answers: The NIH Trial of EDTA Chelation Therapy."

3. "Questions & Answers: The NIH Trial of EDTA Chelation Therapy for Coronary Artery Disease."

4. Cardiologist James C. Roberts of Toledo, Ohio who in past has tried chelation therapy and vitamin therapy with patients, summarizes this view in a message to the authors, stating, "we know that IV and vitamin C confers tremendous benefits; just 1000 mg a day of vitamin C decreases 10 year event rate by 43 percent." Fax to the authors April 2, 2003.

5. E. Cranton, A. Brecher J. Frackleton, *Bypassing Bypass: A Non-Surgical Therapy for Improving Circulation and Slowing the Aging Process* (Hampton Roads, Va: Medex Inc., 1980).

6. April Quinones, "EDTA Chelation and Calcium," [online], http://www.anitafinley.com/sept00/calcium.html; see also "Magnesium EDTA, Chelation for Life," 2002 [online], http://www.chelationforlife.com/Faqs/magnesium2.html [March 31, 2003].

7. Todd J. Anderson, Jaroslav Hubacek, D. George Wyse, Merril L. Knudtson, "Effect of Chelation Therapy on Endothelial Function in Patients with Coronary Artery Disease: PATCH Substudy," *Journal of the American College of Cardiology (JACC)* 41, Issue 3 (February 5, 2003): 420-25. This study basically says that chelation therapy has no measurable positive impacts on patients with heart disease.

8. Ibid. Chelation therapists have vociferously rebutted the study. See Elmer Cranton, "Dr. Cranton's Rebuttal Of the JAMA Article on IV Chelation Therapy," Chelation Therapy [online], http:/

ww.chelationtherapyonline.com/articles/p209.htm [April 15, 2003].

9. Saul Green, Wallace Sampson, "EDTA Chelation Therapy for Atherosclerosis And Degenerative Diseases: Implausibility and Paradoxical Oxidant Effects," [online], http://ww.quackwatch.org /01QuackeryRelatedTopics/chelationimp.html [March 30, 2003], quoting: Anon. AMA Council on Scientific Affairs: chelation therapy, *JAMA* 250, 5 (1983): 672.

10. "Questions & Answers: The NIH Trial of EDTA Chelation Therapy for Coronary Artery Disease."

11. Ibid.

12. Interview with Gary Mezo, Tampa, Florida, October 16, 2002.

13. Interview with Gary Mezo, October 16, 2002 and comments added February 15, 2003.

14. Interviews by the authors in late 2002 and early 2003 with James C. Roberts and other physicians who prescribe the nanobiotic therapy.

15. Correspondence by James C. Roberts to the authors, April 2, 2003.

16. Shiels *et al.*, "Treatment of Lead Poisoning by Edathamil Calcium-Disodium." Also, "Questions & Answers: The NIH Trial of EDTA Chelation Therapy for Coronary Artery Disease."

17. Note from Gary Mezo to the authors, February 16, 2003.

18. Interviews with Neva Çiftçíoglu and Olavi Kajander, October 2002 through February 2003, based on their unpublished investigations.

19. N. Çiftçíoglu, M. A. Miller-Hjelle, J. T. Hjelle, and E. O. Kajander, "Inhibition of Nanobacteria by Antimicrobial Drugs as Measured by a Modified Microdilution Method," *Antimicrobial Agents and Chemotherapy* 46, no. 7 (July 2002): 2077-86 [online], http://aac.asm.org/cgi/content/full/46/7/2077?maxtoshow=&HITS =10&hits=10&RESULTFORMAT=&titleabstract=nano-bacteria&searchid=1043171003292 7860&stored search =&FIRSTINDEX=0&search url=http%3A%2F%2F journals.asm.org%2Fcgi%2Fsearch [January 21, 2003].

20. "Noncompliance results in an estimated 125,000 deaths a year from cardiovascular disease alone, up to a quarter of nursing home admissions and an estimated 10% of hospital admissions." Delia O'Hara, "Given But Not Taken: When Your Patients Don't Take Their Medicines," *American Medical News*, Feb. 4, 2002 [online], http://www.ama-assn.org/sci-pubs/amnews/pick 02/ hlsa0204.htm [March 31, 2003].

Chapter 10 Does It Work?

1.   R. G. H., letter to NanobacLabs, February 11, 2002.

2.   Excerpts from hand-written testimonials sent to NanobacLabs Jan.-Mar., 2003.

3.   Interview with Dr. C. April 10, 2003.

4.   James C. Roberts Jr., "Overview," heartfixer.com [online], http://www.heartfixer.com/overview.htm [December 29, 2002].

5.   Correspondence from Dr. James C. Roberts to the authors, April 2, 2003.

6.   James C. Roberts Jr., "*Nanobacterium sanguineum* Home Page," heartfixer.com [online], http://www.heartfixer.com/indexNB.htm [December 29, 2002]. Roberts has cited NanobacLabs's first in-house study of the impacts of NanobacTX on heart disease patients.

7.   On the www.heartfixer.com website, there is a subsection entitled "*Nanobacterium sanguineum*."

8.   www.heartfixer.com/NB - Case Studies.htm [April 15, 2003].

9.   James C. Roberts Jr., "# 2 MP: NanobacTX for Atherosclerosis Everywhere," Patient Case Study [online], http://www.heartfixer.com/NB%20%20Case%20Studies.htm##1MP:%20%20NanobacTX%20for%20atherosclerosis%20everywhere [March 30, 2003].

10. www.heartfixer.com/NB - Case Studies.htm

11. Ibid.

12. Ibid.

13. Ibid.

14. Correspondence from Dr. James C. Roberts Jr. to the authors, April 2, 2003.

15. James C. Roberts Jr., "#15 MJ: The Up-Down Phenomena," Patient Case Study [online], http://www.heartfixer.com/NB%20%20Case%20Studies.htm##15%20MJ:%20%20The%20Up-Down%20Phenomena [March 30, 2003].

16. Interview by the authors with Dr. Maniscalco, Tampa, Florida, October 16, 2002.

17. Ibid.

18. In 1997 at least 44,000 patients died from medical errors in the U.S. according to: Linda T. Kohn, Janet M. Corrigan, Molla S. Donaldson, editors, *To Err Is Human: Building a Safer Health System,* Institute of Medicine, (Washington, D.C.: National Acad-

emy Press, 1999.) This data has been disputed, but its authoritative source suggests that medical error especially in prescribing drugs is a problem.

19. D. M. Eisenberg, R. B. Davis, S. Ettner, S. Appel, S. Wilkey, M. Van Rompay, R. C. Kessler, "Trends in Alternative Medicine Use in the United States 1990-97: Results of a Follow-up National Survey," *JAMA* 280 (1998): 1569-75.

20. Nancy Keates, "The Holistic Hospital," *Wall Street Journal* (March 28, 2003): W1.

21. Tinker Ready, "Trials Suspended Due to Death at Hopkins," *Nature Medicine* 7, no. 8 (August 2001): 877 [online], http://www.nature.com/cgi-taf/DynaPage.taf?file=/nm/journal/v7/n8/full/m0801_877b.html [January 21, 2003].

22. The Western IRB is not a testing agency, but rather sets the ground rules for studies on new treatments. Its mission is to "Protect the Rights and Welfare of the Human Research Subject." It is the oldest and most experienced independent IRB in America. The Board has reviewed research by more than 10,000 investigators in over 30 countries, and in every U.S. state. Western IRB Website [online], http://www.wirb.com/ [January 21, 2003].

23. Interview with Dr. Maniscalco, October 16, 2002.

24. Ibid.

25. Ibid.

26. The clinical trial study paper is entitled "Nanobacteria: Stealthy Pathogen in Atherogenesis, Results from the NanobacTX-ACESII Cardiology Study: A Novel Nanobiotic for the Reduction of Calcified Plaque" (in submission). Other comments in this section are taken from interviews with Dr. Maniscalco, October 16, 2002, and March 19, 2003.

27. Interview with Dr. Maniscalco, October 16, 2002.

28. Ibid.

29. Interview with J. K., October 31, 2002.

30. Interview with Dr. C. April 10, 2003.

Chapter 11 Caution...

1. This quote from Dr. Roberts's website was modified as a result of correspondence with Dr. Roberts, April 2, 2003. See www.heartfixer.com for more information. Dr. Roberts has used NanobacTX in combination with Enhanced External Counter

Pulsation (EECP), a therapy to help the body naturally bypass blocked arteries.

2.   Rauno Harvima, "Association of Nanobacteria with Dermato-logical Diseases," NanobacLabs website [online], http://www.NanobacLabs.com/NanobacLabs-nanobacteria-current-research.asp [April 26, 2003].

3.   "The Jarisch-Herxheimer reaction describes the release of en-dotoxin when large numbers of organisms are killed by antibiot-ics." Jarisch-Herxheimer reaction, General Practice Notebook—a UK medical encyclopedia on the world wide web http://www.gpnotebook.co.uk/cache/2140798985.htm

4.   M. Y. Rabau, M. Baratz, P. Rozen, "Na2 Ethylenediamine-tetraacetic Acid Retention Enema in Dogs: Biochemical and His-tological Response," General Pharmacology 22, no. 2 (1991): 329-30.

5.   Interviews by the authors with Drs. Maniscalco, Roberts, and other physicians between October 2002 and May 2003.

6.   A Nanobac-TX ACES Clinical Study carried out by NanobacLabs (now Nanobac Pharmaceuticals) showed decreases in coronary artery calcification, with EBCT scores reduced by an average of 58 percent, according to: Kajander *et al.*, "The Pathogenesis of Vascular Calcification," Poster session, Tampere, Finland, Feb-ruary 21, 2003. Dr. James C. Roberts and Dr. Benedict Maniscalco indicated to the authors in various interviews in March and April 2003 that such high percentage reduction had not been achieved with their patients in the same four-month period. None-theless, they added that calcium scores often began to fall dra-matically if the patients continued for more time. The treatment timeframe and conditions of patients seem key. More will be learned about this as additional studies occur.

7.   *The Sinatra Health Report*, the monthly subscription newsletter of Stephen Sinatra, M.D., F.A.C.C., June '02 issue.

Chapter 12 Who Pays...

1.   Janelle Carter, "Health Care Spending Jumps 8.7 Percent," *Asso-ciated Press*, January 8, 2003, reporting on the annual report of the Centers for Medicare and Medicaid. And "Survey: Health insurance premiums up 14 percent," *Houston Business Journal*, September 11, 2003 [online], http://www.bizjournals.com/houston/stories/2003/09/08/daily37.html [September 11, 2003].

2.   Patient-Directed-Care   website   [online],   http://www.patientdirectedcare.com [January 23, 2003].

3.   Telephone interview by the authors with Dr. Alan Iezzi, October 16, 2002.

4. "FDA Moves to Shut Down Canada Drug Broker," *Associated Press, New York Times*, September 17, 2003 [online], http://www.nytimes.com/aponline/national/AP-Canada-Drugs.html?pagewanted=print&position= [September 17, 2003].

5. Telephone interview by the authors with Dr. Alan Iezzi, October 16, 2002.

6. "Medical Malpractice Insurance: Stable Losses/Unstable Rates," Americans For Insurance Reform, New York, October 10, 2002: "Not only has there been no real increase [of] lawsuits, jury awards or any tort system costs at any time during the last three decades, but the astronomical premium increases that some doctors have been charged during periodic insurance "crises" over this time period are in exact sync with the economic cycle of the insurance industry, driven by interest rates and investments."

7. Telephone interview by the authors with Dr. Alan Iezzi, October 16, 2002.

8. Joanna L. Krotz, "Check Out The Revolution In Health Care," bCentral, August 2003 [online], http://www.bcentral.com/articles/krotz/140.asp [August 1, 2003].

9. Bruce Japsen, "Medical Insurance Directed By Users," *Chicago Tribune*, December 27, 2002 [online], http://www.sltrib.com/2002/Dec/12272002/Business/14815.asp [August 1, 2003].

10. Nancy Keates, "The Holistic Hospital," *Wall Street Journal* (March 28, 2003): W1.

11. This list was provided in an email to the authors from NanobacLabs, January 15, 2003, and in a fax September 12, 2003.

12. Healthcare for indigent persons is one of America's most persistent socio-economic problems. "In 1991 Hillsborough county commissioner Phyllis Busansky spearheaded a drive in Hillsborough County to create a primary health care program for the indigent and working poor." "UTMB Health Policy Lecture to Focus on Indigent Care Plan," Press Release, University of Texas Medical Branch at Galveston 2000 [online], http://www.utmb.edu/utmbnews/00pr_archive/HPF0600.htm [January 23, 2003]. "…About 19,000 poor and low-income people are enrolled in the plan, which uses 12 primary care clinics, five hospitals and 600 physicians. The plan has served as a national model for its funding and breadth. It has saved the county an estimated $100 million in emergency medical bills for people who otherwise couldn't afford to see doctors before their conditions become dire and more expensive. The county's indigent health care plan was created in 1991 and funded with an annual $26 million in property taxes and a half-cent sales tax. By 1997, the fund was so flush, commissioners eliminated the property tax supplement and cut the sales tax to a quarter-cent. But by November 2000, the fund

was getting low. By a previous agreement, the sales tax will return to a half-cent again next month, but that won't be enough...."
Kathryn Wexler, "Health Care Cuts Reconsidered," *St. Petersburg Times* September 7, 2001 [online], http://www.sptimes.com/News/090701/TampaBay/Health_care_cuts_reco.shtml [January 23, 2003].

Chapter 13 What We Know...

1. The link between nanobacteria, periodontal disease, and atherosclerosis was recently strengthened by Neva Çíftçíoglu in a letter to *Circulation*, the journal of the American College of Cardiology, in which she identifies nanobacteria as the one pathogen that dentists may have failed to detect when atempting to find the link between tooth extraction and subsequent heart problems in their patients. N. Çiftçioglu, D.S. McKay, E.O. Kajander, "Association Between Nanobacteria and Periodontal Disease," *Circulation* 108 (August 2003): 58-9. This, combined with Kajander's new work on nanobacteria binding prothrombin may explain why many patients experience heart problems associated with thrombosis after a tooth extraction (personal communication from E. Olavi Kajander to the authors, May 2003).

2. For updates go to www.calcify.com.

Milestones

1. R. L. Folk, "SEM Imaging of Bacteria and Nannobacteria in Carbonate Sediments and Rocks," *Journal of Sedimentary Petrology* 63 (1993): 990-99.

2. E. Olavi Kajander, "Culture and Detection Method for Sterile-Filterable Autonomously Replicating Biological Particles," *US Patent No 5,135,851* 16 pp., 1992.

3. E. O. Kajander, E. Tahvanainen, I. Kuronen, N. Çiftçioglu, "Comparison of Staphylococci and Novel Bacteria-like Particles from Blood," Abstract, 7th International Symposium on Staphylococci and Staphylococcal Infections, June 29-July 3, 1992, Stockholm, Abstract book, p. 79, 1992. Also, K. Ackerman, I. Kuronen, E. O. Kajander, "Scanning Electron Microscopy of Nanobacteria-Novel Biofilm Producing Organisms in Blood," *Scanning* 15 (1993): III.

4. D. S. McKay , E. K. Gibson Jr., K. L. Thomas-Keprta , H. Vali, C. S. Romanek, S. J. Clemett., X.D.F. Chillier, C.R. Maechling, and R.N. Zare, "Search for Past Life on Mars: Possible Relic Biogenic Activity in Martian Meteorite ALH 84001," *Science* 273 (Aug. 16, 1996): 924-30.

5. N. Çiftçioglu, I. Kuronen, K. Åkerman, E. Hiltunen, J. Laukkanen, E. O. Kajander, "A New Potential Threat in Antigen and Antibody Products: Nanobacteria," In: *Vaccines 97* eds. F. Brown, D. Burton, P. Doherty, J. Mekalanos, E. Norrby (Cold Spring Harbor: Spring Harbor Laboratory Press, 1997), 99-103.

6. K. K. Åkerman, J. T. Kuikka, N. Çiftçioglu, J. Parkkinen, K. A. Bergström, I. Kuronen, E. O. Kajander, "Radiolabeling and In Vivo Distribution of Nanobacteria in Rabbit," *Proceedings SPIE* 3111 (1997): 436-42.

7. E. O. Kajander, N. Çiftçioglu, "Nanobacteria: An Alternative Mechanism for Pathogenic Intra- and Extracellular Mineralisation and Stone Formation," *Proceedings of the National Academy of Sciences* (1995): 8274-79.

8. N. Çiftçioglu, V. Çiftçioglu, H. Vali, E. Turcott, E. O. Kajander, "Sedimentary Rocks in our Mouth: Dental Pulp Stones Made by Nanobacteria," *Proceedings SPIE* 3441 (1998): 130-35.

9. E. Garcia-Cuerpo; E. O. Kajander, N. Çiftçioglu, F. L. Castellano, C. Correa, J. Conzales, F. Mampaso, F. Liano, E. G. de Gabiola and Y. A .E. Berrilero, "Nanobacteria. Un Modelo de Neo-litogenesis Experimental," *Arch. Esp. Urol.* 53(4) (2000): 291-303.

10. J. T. Hjelle, M. A. Miller-Hjelle, I. R. Poxton, O. Kajander, N. Çiftçioglu, M. L. Jones, R. C. Caughey, R. Brown, P. D. Millikin, F. S. Darras, "Endotoxin and Nanobacteria in Polycystic Kidney Disease," *Kidney International* 57 (2000): 2360-74.

11. E. Olavi Kajander, Neva Çiftçioglu, Katja Aho, "Detection of Nanobacteria in Viral Vaccines," Proceedings of the American Society for Microbiology, 101st General Meeting of the American Society for Microbiology (May 2-24, 2001), Abstract Y-3, p. 736. Michael Le Page, "The Tiny Villains Lurking in Vaccines," *New Scientist* 170, 2293 (June 3, 2001): 12.

12. Rasmussen *et al.*, "Electron Microscope and Immunological Evidence of Nanobacterial-Like Structures," *JACC* 39, issue 5 (6 March 2002): Supplement A.

13. Neva Çiftçioglu, "Risk for Nanobacteria in Gamma Globulin Preparations," 102nd General Meeting of the American Society for Microbiology.

14. Martin Kerner, Heinz Hohenberg, Siegmund Ertl, Marcus Reckermann, Alejandro Spitzy, "Self-organization of Dissolved Organic Matter to Micelle-like Microparticles in River Water," *Nature* 422 (March 13, 2003): 150-54.

15. B. Maniscalco, "Shouldering the Risk Burden," *Circulation* (March 25, 2003).

16. Kajander *et al.*, "The Pathogenesis Of Vascular Calcification," Poster session, Tampere, Finland, February 21, 2003.

17. Garcia-Cuerpo *et al.*, "Nanobacteria. Un Modelo de Neo-litogenesis Experimental." Also E. Garcia-Cuerpo, E. O. Kajander, "Litogenesis. Hacia un nuevo planteamiento," *Arch. Esp. Urol.* 54(9) (2001): 851-53.

Glossary

1. "Calcium Scan Predicts Heart Attack Risk in Physically Fit People," American Heart Association News Release, January 3, 2001 [online], http://www.americanheart.org/presenter.jhtml?identifier=3292 [April 3, 2003].

2. Uffe Ravnskov, "The Cholesterol Myths: Exposing the Fallacy that Saturated Fat and Cholesterol Cause Heart Disease," NewTrends Publishing, Inc. 2000. Excerpts found at [online], http://www.heart-disease-bypass-surgery.com/data/articles/36.htm#references [April 5, 2003].

3. "CRP Improves Cardiovascular Risk Prediction in Metabolic Syndrome, Circulation," *Journal of the American Heart Association*, January 1, 2003 [online], http://www.americanheart.org/presenter.jhtml?identifier=3007985 [April 3, 2003].

4. "Computer Imaging / Tomography," American Heart Association [online], http://www.americanheart.org/presenter.jhtml?identifier=4554#ct [April 3, 2003].

5. "Fibrinogen," Medline Plus, National Library of Medicine, November 25, 2001 [online], http://www.nlm.nih.gov/medlineplus/ency/article/03650.htm [April 5, 2003].

6. "What Is High Blood Pressure?" National Heart, Lung, and Blood Institute, NIH [online], http://www.nhlbi.nih.gov/hbp/hbp/whathbp.htm [April 5, 2003].

7. "What Is Nutrition?" Study Guide, University of Utah, Division of Foods and Nutrition [online], http://www.health.utah.edu/fdnu/1020-001-020StudyGuide2.htm [April 5, 2003].

8. "MRI," Medline Plus, National Library of Medicine, November 28, 2001 [online], http://www.nlm.nih.gov/medlineplus/ency/article/003335.htm [April 4, 2003].

9. M. L. Knudtson, D. G. Wyse, P. D. Galbraith *et al.*, "Chelation Therapy for Ischemic Heart Disease. A Randomized Controlled Trial," *JAMA* 287 (2002): 481-86. Abstract found [online], http://www.ccs.ca/society/congress2002/abstracts/abs/a260.htm [April 5, 2003].

10. "ESR," Medline Plus, National Library of Medicine, November 23, 2001 [online], http://www.nlm.nih.gov/medlineplus/ency/article/003638.htm [April 5, 2003].

11. "Drug to Lower Cholesterol Also Slows Calcium Build-up in Arteries," Journal Report, American Heart Association, February 8, 2002 [online], http://www.Americanheart.org/presenter.jhtml;jsessionid=2RZC0OMO5WABBWFZOAGSCZQ?identifier=3004052 [April 3, 2003].

Who's Who In The World Of Calcification And Nanobacteria

1. R.Y. Morita, "Bioavailability of Energy and Starvation Survival in Nature," Canadian Journal of Microbiology 34 (1988): 436-41.

2. R.Y. Morita, *Bacteria in Oligotrophic Environments - Starvation-Survival Life Styles* (Dordrecht, Netherlands: Kluwer Academic Publishers, 1997).

INDEX

This is the index for the main body of the book. To avoid repetition, it excludes names of many individuals described in the Who's Who appendix, and some of the technical terms described in the Glossary. Please refer to those sections for alphabetically indexed information.

A

About The Authors

Douglas Mulhall's previous book, *Our Molecular Future*, co-researched by Katja Hansen, was selected by New Scientist magazine for its "must-read" list, featured in bestseller lists of Barnes & Noble and Amazon.com, and chosen as a finalist in the Independent Publishers Book Award Science category. It has been praised by numerous other organizations such as the Foresight Institute, and the Association of College & Research Libraries who chose it as an Outstanding Academic Title. Libraries around the world now carry the book, which is described further at www.OurMolecularFuture.com.

Mulhall's journalistic and Hansen's biological engineering backgrounds are supported by years of experience managing the disease prevention and environmental science programs of international scientific research institutes. They have co-founded and managed European and South American organizations devoted to research and communications. Their experience with preventing microbiological infections comes from pioneering water purification technologies in collaboration with multinational chemicals companies and multilateral government agencies. The systems are now being replicated on three continents.

Other works of Mulhall and Hansen show how technology convergence is transforming our lives in everything from water recycling to world expositions. Their articles are published by *Financial Times*, *Newsday*, *National Post*, *The Futurist*, *Futures Research Quarterly*, *Frankfurter Allgemeine Zeitung*, *Water, Environment and Technology*, National Research Council, and the Center for Responsible Nanotechnology, to mention a few.

To get updates make sure to visit

www.calcify.com

the website for this book!

Quick Order Form

☏ Fax Orders: 561-630-0375. Send this form.

☎ Telephone Orders: Call 800-245-2133 toll free.

🖳 Email Orders: order@calcify.com

✉ Postal Orders: 21st Century Eloquence, 7108 Fairway Dr., Suite 101, Palm Beach Gardens, FL 33418

I herewith order:

Has Heart Disease Been Cured?

[Suggested Retail Price $ 17.95 plus S&H*]

Number of copies:_____

Name:_____

Address:_____

City:_____

Postal Code:_____

Country:_____

Telephone:_____

E-Mail address:_____

☐ Check if shipping address is same as billing address, otherwise complete below:

Shipping Address:_____

City:_____

Postal Code:_____

Country:_____

Payment:

☐Visa ☐Mastercard ☐American Express ☐Discover

Card Number:_____

Name on card:_____ Exp. Date:_____

* Shipping charges vary depending on destination. Airmail: approx. $9.00. For courier deliveries please contact customer service at sales@voicerecognition.com. All charges are in U.S. Dollars.